Understanding Payment for Advanced Practice Nursing Services

Volume One: Medicare Reimbursement

Sheila Abood, MS, RN

Associate Director, Government Affairs

American Nurses Association

David Keepnews, JD, MPH, RN, FAAN

Assistant Professor, Department of Health and Clinical Sciences

University of Massachusetts Lowell

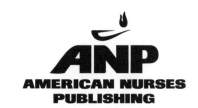

ANP

AMERICAN NURSES PUBLISHING

WASHINGTON, D.C.

Library of Congress Cataloging-in-Publication Data

Abood, Sheila
    Understanding payment for advanced practice nursing services / Sheila Abood, David Keepnews.
       208 p. ; 1.3 cm.
    Includes bibliographical references.
    Contents: v. 1. Medicare reimbursement.
    ISBN 1-55810-148-9
    1. Nurse practitioners —Fees—United States. 2. Health insurance claims—United States.
    3. Medicare. 4. Medicaid. I. Keepnews, David. II. American Nurses Association. III. Title.
    [DNLM: 1. Nursing Services—economics. 2. Reimbursement Mechanisms—
    organization & administration. 3. Medicaid. 4. Medicare. 5. Nurse Clinicians.
    6. Nurse Practitioners. WY 77 A154u 2000]
    RT82.8+
    331.2'81362173--dc21
    00-033187

The material in this publication is intended to provide the reader with general information about Medicare Part B payment policies and procedures. It is not intended as specific advice about individual billing matters or legal advice, and should not be relied upon as such. Readers should contact an appropriate billing professional or service for advice or assistance regarding billing Medicare for health care services.

Published by

American Nurses Publishing

600 Maryland Avenue, SW

Suite 100 West

Washington, DC 20024-2571

ISBN 1-55810-148-9

APNS-20   2M   11/00

Contents

INTRODUCTION

January 1, 1998, was a day of tremendous significance for nursing. On that day, Section 4511 of Public Law 105-33—the Balanced Budget Act (BBA) of 1997—became law. This section of the BBA expanded Medicare coverage of services provided by nurse practitioners (NPs) and clinical nurse specialists (CNSs). Although NP and CNS services had been covered in limited settings for several years, the new law provided for Medicare coverage regardless of geographic area or practice setting. The new law dramatically expanded the ability of NPs and CNSs to meet the health care needs of Medicare beneficiaries in communities around the country. The passage of this law was, unquestionably, a big victory for nurses and health care consumers alike.

This change also means that many NPs and CNSs are, or soon will be, dealing with a sea of legal, regulatory, and bureaucratic requirements that apply to professionals who participate in the Medicare program. These clinicians will need to know how to enroll as Medicare providers, what kinds of services are covered, how much they will get paid for their services, what special legal or other requirements are imposed on their services as NPs and CNSs, where to direct questions, and so on. After listening to their physician colleagues complain for years about the "hassle factor" involved in Medicare (and other) reimbursement, NPs and CNSs now get to share in that experience as well.

But nurses have had ample experience in dealing with bureaucratic, legal, and institutional barriers and in navigating those barriers to ensure their patients the best, highest quality care possible. To do so, nurses need the right tools. They need to know what rules apply. They need to know how to change the rules that get in the way of providing care. This experience is, after all, what nurses used in winning Medicare coverage of NP and CNS services in the first place and in removing geographic and practice barriers from reimbursement through the change in the law in 1997.

In 1993, American Nurses Publishing produced *The Reimbursement Manual: How to Get Paid for Your Advanced Practice Nursing Services* (Mittelstadt 1993). That book gave NPs and CNSs the tools to understand a range of reimbursement options. It also provided source material, including applicable federal regulations and laws, to understand the rules that applied to those options. Since 1993, the rules have changed significantly, and nurses are in need of a means to understand and access the laws, regulations, and policies that govern their ability to provide patient care services and to be reimbursed appropriately for those services.

The need for this new volume is made particularly pressing by the expansion of Medicare reimbursement. However, nurses' ability to understand how to get paid for their services is by no means limited to Medicare. For that reason, the present volume is the first in a series on NP and CNS reimbursement that will cover Medicare, Medicaid, other government-sponsored reimbursement programs, and private insurance programs. More in-depth information will be provided on aspects of the Medicare program, such as the processes by which services are coded and valued under the Medicare Fee Schedule as well as fraud and abuse issues. Some initial discussion of these topics is included in this volume.

The goal of this first volume is to provide NPs and CNSs with some of the basics of Medicare reimbursement, including an understanding of the Medicare program and the laws, rules, and policies that govern it, as well as an introduction to the specifics of billing for NP and CNS services.

It is hoped that the present publication will provide a useful tool for NPs and CNSs as they seek to expand their ability to provide high-quality, sensitive, competent services to greater numbers of patients. That goal has been foremost in working for and winning reimbursement for NPs and CNSs from the start. If this publication helps in realizing that goal, it will be a source of considerable satisfaction for the authors.

Sheila Abood, MS, RN

Washington, D.C.

David Keepnews, JD, MPH, RN, FAAN

Lowell, MA

OVERVIEW OF MEDICARE

Introduction and Background

This book provides nurse practitioners (NPs) and clinical nurse specialists (CNSs) with the tools necessary to understand Medicare payment for their services and how to bill the Medicare program for services they provide to Medicare beneficiaries. The book will also be useful to others who are interested in NP and CNS services under Medicare—from office and hospital billing personnel to educators to NP and CNS students. The authors believe that NPs and CNSs will benefit not only from a how-to approach to Medicare billing but also from a basic understanding of the Medicare program itself and of where their services fit into that program. Although the billing process itself may largely revolve around completing and filing forms, the more that NPs and CNSs understand about the context in which their services are provided (and paid for), the more they will be able to exercise professional judgment and critical thinking in maximizing beneficiaries' access to their services.

Medicare and Medicaid

The Medicare and Medicaid programs were initiated in 1965 as a result of congressional action. Both programs were the result of efforts over many years to increase health care coverage for underserved Americans. Both programs were created by amending the Social Security Act. Medicare is sometimes referred to as *Title 18* because the laws governing that program are contained in Title 18 of the Social Security Act. Medicaid is often referred to as *Title 19* because the laws governing it are found in Title 19 of the Social Security Act.

Medicare and Medicaid are two separate programs that target two different populations. Medicare provides coverage for virtually all Americans age 65 years and older, the permanently disabled, and patients with end-stage renal disease.

Medicaid provides health care coverage for many of the poor. Medicaid operates as a joint federal–state partnership. It is funded by both federal and state moneys. The federal laws and regulations provide a basic framework for Medicaid, including mandates for basic services, eligibility, and appeal rights. Each state administers its own Medicaid program within this framework and has the option of adding on to it by providing services and covering individuals beyond those required by the federal government. Federal law requires Medicaid to cover services of certified family NPs and certified pediatric NPs, as well as certified nurse-midwives. Some states have opted to cover services of all NPs (as opposed to only family and pediatric NPs), and some cover the services of CNSs (or of some types of CNSs, such as psychiatric–mental health CNSs).

Unlike Medicaid, Medicare is exclusively a federal program. Federal law defines the structure of the program, including benefits and coverage. For the most part, states do not have a direct role in shaping the Medicare program.

1

Medicare Part A and Part B

Medicare consists of two main parts that operate virtually as two separate programs. Medicare Part A, also known as Hospital Insurance, covers hospitalization, skilled nursing facility (SNF) services, and some home health services. Medicare Part B, also known as Supplemental Medical Insurance, covers services of physicians and other practitioners, outpatient hospital services, laboratory procedures, medical equipment, and additional home health expenses. Part A is financed by a payroll tax of 1.45 percent levied on both employers and employees. Part B is financed by a combination of premiums paid by beneficiaries (in 2000, premiums were $45.50 a month) and by general fund (i.e., tax) revenues.

It is Medicare Part B that pays for non-institutional services provided by NPs and CNSs and will, thus, be the main focus of this book.

Physician Services under Part B

As a result of the 1997 changes in the law, Medicare covers certain services provided by NPs and CNSs. The law states that, under defined circumstances, services provided by NPs and CNSs will be considered *physicians' services*. It is important from the outset to understand why and how this term is used under Medicare. Some NPs and CNSs may find it confusing or even bothersome to be told that they are paid when their services qualify as physicians' services, whereas others may have no problem with this at all.

It is critical to remember that the Medicare program as a whole is based on a medical model. Part B was designed in 1965 as a source of payment for services provided by physicians to elderly patients. The program continues to reflect this orientation. It is a program of medical insurance that covers physicians' services. To the extent that services of other practitioners are covered, it is because the law provides either that some practitioners may (under some circumstances) be considered "physicians" or that the services of certain practitioners will be considered physicians' services.

Medicare law does not recognize or cover nurse practitioner services or clinical nurse specialist services as such. It covers physicians' services when provided by physicians and, when other conditions are met, when provided by other specified practitioners, including NPs and CNSs. This distinction may appear semantic and, in practice, may not be a significant one for many NPs and CNSs, depending on the kind of services they provide.

Although the term *physicians' services* is a term of art and is the term primarily used in Medicare law, the terms *Part B services* and *professional services* are often used in Medicare rules and policies. The three terms are used interchangeably.

Benefits and Services under Part B

The fact that Part B covers physicians' services does not mean that every service provided by a physician is covered. Part B covers services related to the treatment of active medical problems: A patient goes to his or her physician for treatment of diabetes, a patient goes to a clinic complaining of joint pain, or a patient is visited in the hospital by his or her physician after being hospitalized with a myocardial infarction. Medicare has not historically included coverage for many important preventive services and screenings. This coverage has changed somewhat in recent years, because Congress has added coverage for more screening services. However, some basic elements of preventive care, such as regular physical examinations for well patients or education and outreach activities designed to maintain health, are not covered. Although the nursing profession has advocated shifting Medicare from a medical model to one that focuses on wellness and prevention, the program remains focused on a primarily medical, illness-oriented model.

Direct and Indirect Medicare Payments

Medicare payment to NPs and CNSs is a relatively recent development. Coverage of services (or some of the services) of NPs and CNSs is not.

The mechanism for coverage of services provided by NPs and CNSs that was added to Medicare law as a result of the 1997 law is sometimes referred to as *direct reimbursement*. This term is used because it involves recognition of those services and the availability of payment being made directly to the NP or CNS. It stands in contrast to other mechanisms that are sometimes referred to as *indirect reimbursement*. (This term is not an official Medicare term but is rather a description that has been used by nurses and nursing organizations.) Indirect reimbursement has generally meant that services are covered as part of payment that goes to someone else, such as a physician, who may then pay the NP or CNS. (This payment may be based on the income the physician derives from NP or CNS services or on a salary that may or may not take into account the income that these services produce.)

The chief example of indirect reimbursement is referred to as *incident to* payment. Medicare covers (among other things) services and supplies that are furnished incident to a physicians' professional services. This broad category has been part of the Medicare program since its inception. It was really not intended as a mechanism for providing reimbursement for services provided by nonphysician practitioners; rather, it recognized that some employees of the physician provide some reimbursable services by acting, essentially, as an extra set of hands for the physician. "Incident to" payment is made to the physician, as if he or she performed the service himself or herself.

This arrangement did not envision the development of NP or CNS practice or a growth in the autonomy of professional nursing practice. It involved an entirely dependent relationship, intended to pay for services of employees of the physician acting as an extension of the physician.

"Incident to" payment also comes with a number of important restrictions. "Incident to" services must be an integral but an incidental part of the physician's service, is commonly rendered without charge or included in the physician's bill, is of a type commonly furnished in physicians' offices or in clinics, is furnished under the physician's direct personal supervision, and is furnished by an employee of the physician (*Medicare Carriers Manual* Section 2050). These conditions are further interpreted to mean that the physician must be physically present and

3

available in the office suite where services are provided (although not necessarily present in the same room where services are provided) (*Medicare Carriers Manual* Section 2050.1). Many Medicare carriers had also concluded that, for services to qualify for incident to payment, the physician must have initiated the patient's treatment (i.e., that the NP or CNS could not be the patient's first point of contact).

Over time, this arrangement became more and more untenable for many NPs and CNSs. Although NPs and CNSs were being used to provide coverage in an office, "incident to" payment meant that services could not be covered if no physician was present, for example, when the physician took a day off, went to see hospitalized patients, or took a lunch break (unless another physician remained on the premises). It meant that NPs and CNSs could not perform house calls unless a physician went along. In many practice settings, "incident to" situations became more and more problematic because the arrangements required for payment failed to reflect current professional practice.

Historical Perspectives on Medicare Coverage of NP and CNS Services

Although the authors do not anticipate that most readers will have great historical interest in the details of Medicare coverage issues prior to the passage of the Balanced Budget Act (BBA) of 1997, some familiarity with the evolution of coverage of NP and CNS services provides some useful context for understanding the current status of coverage and of some continuing issues related to payment for NP and CNS services.

1965–1989

At the start of the Medicare program, no provision was made for payment to nurses of any sort for providing physicians' services. This fact is probably not surprising, considering that few nurses functioned as independently practicing clinicians in 1965. Services provided by nurses in physicians' offices and in clinics were covered, if at all, as services provided incident to those of a physician. This "incident to" provision is explained in detail in the section "Direct and Indirect Medicare Payments."

1989

The Omnibus Budget Reconciliation Act of 1989 (OBRA '89) contained two important provisions related to payment for NP services. One provision required Medicaid coverage for services of certified family NPs and certified pediatric NPs. Another provided for Medicare Part B coverage for services provided by NPs in skilled nursing facilities (SNFs). Those provisions were an important advance in recognizing the ability of NPs to provide necessary services for patients, particularly geriatric patients. It also established, for the first time, Medicare payment for services provided by NPs. However, payment was restricted to only one practice setting, the SNF. It was also limited to NPs; it did not cover services provided by CNSs. Moreover, the law provided that payment for NP services was to go to the NP's employer, not to the NP.

1990

The following year, OBRA '90 included an important provision establishing Medicare coverage of Part B services provided by NPs and CNSs in rural areas. This provision was a significant step forward in establishing NPs and CNSs as Medicare providers. Its direct effect was limited in scope, however. The legislation targeted rural areas in an effort to increase access to health care providers in underserved areas in which physicians were often in short supply.

In practice, however, coverage did not extend to all rural areas. The new law defined "rural area" as one other than a metropolitan statistical area (MSA) county, in other words, a non-MSA county. Many counties may include rural portions within them or even be primarily rural yet also include a city or be close enough to a city to be considered an MSA county. Because OBRA '90 used the MSA and non-MSA distinction, services provided by NPs and CNSs in mixed urban and rural counties could not be covered by Medicare. It was not uncommon to hear from NPs or CNSs practicing in areas surrounded by farmland and dirt roads whose services were considered ineligible for Medicare coverage because an urban area located several hours away in the same county rendered it an MSA county.

Still, the significance of OBRA '90 should not be downplayed. Many NPs and CNSs were able to begin billing for their services, providing much-needed access to underserved patients and gaining important experience in dealing with Medicare billing procedures. This experience provided an important source of knowledge about Medicare billing for NPs and CNSs and helped to begin educating many Medicare carriers about NP and CNS services. The fact that NPs and CNSs were billing Medicare for their services also provided initial data on Medicare claims filed by those providers.

In addition, OBRA '90 established NPs and CNSs as Medicare providers, which led to nursing earning an entrance into several important forums for Medicare payment policy. For instance, nursing has been represented on advisory committees that are established by the American Medical Association (AMA) and that participate in updating the Current Procedural Terminology (CPT) code book and the Medicare Fee Schedule.

1990–1997

From 1990 to 1997, the American Nurses Association (ANA) and other nursing organizations continued to push for direct coverage of NP and CNS services regardless of geographic or practice setting.

- In 1993–1994, President Clinton's health care reform proposals included provisions to expand Medicare coverage of NP services. Alternative reform proposals included similar provisions. Although none of these proposals was ultimately successful, they served to establish broad, bipartisan support for Medicare coverage of NP and CNS services.

- In 1996, the budget bill proposed by the Republican-controlled Congress included a provision for Medicare Part B coverage of NP services. Although the bill was vetoed (for entirely unrelated reasons), the fact that both the Republican Congress and the

Democratic Administration had established a record of support for advanced practice nursing reimbursement gave cause for optimism.

- In 1997, both the president's budget proposal and the budget bill eventually passed by Congress (and signed into law by the president) included a provision for NP and CNS reimbursement. Years of diligent work by nurses had finally paid off: Medicare payment for services provided by NPs and CNSs was finally the law.

Sources of Medicare Law and Policy

Before going into detail on the BBA provisions on NP and CNS reimbursement, it may be helpful to examine the different ways that Medicare policy is formulated and implemented. It is important to understand these sources of Medicare policy, at least in a general way, and to know what kinds of policy changes have occurred, what kinds of changes may occur in the future, and where they may come from.

Federal Statute

Legislation passed by Congress and signed into law by the president provides the initial source of authority for the Medicare program. The program itself came into being as a result of federal legislation passed in 1965. Changes in eligibility and in benefits have also come about as a result of federal legislation. (Recall that Medicare is an exclusively federal program, unlike Medicaid, which is a joint federal–state program, governed by both federal and state legislation.)

Medicare statutes can be found in the Social Security Act and specifically in Title 18 of that act. Specific provisions in the law are usually referred to by their section numbers, for instance, the main provision in Medicare law that addresses NP and CNS reimbursement is Section 1861(s)(2)(K) of the Social Security Act.

To make a change in federal law, Congress must pass a bill. Although Congress considers a large number of bills each year that pertain to the Medicare and Medicaid programs, changes in those programs are usually included in a massive budget bill agreed to by both houses of Congress toward the end of each year. This is in part because Medicare and Medicaid account for a large part of the federal budget and have such a significant effect on that budget. These bills can go by different popular names and are often referred to as the Omnibus Budget Reconciliation Act of the year in which it is passed. For instance, OBRA '87 included major reforms in nursing home regulation; OBRA '89 and OBRA '90 included provisions on NP and CNS reimbursement. The 1997 bill that included removal of geographic and practice setting requirements for NP and CNS reimbursement was known as the Balanced Budget Act of 1997 (because it established a balanced federal budget).

Even though Medicare and Medicaid changes are typically contained in the annual budget bill, proposals for specific changes often start out as individual bills, as, for instance, Medicare reimbursement for NPs and CNSs did. Even though it is usually unlikely that such changes will be passed as individual bills, introducing specific legislation is still an important way to establish and to obtain strong support from members and leaders of both houses of Congress, which, in turn, can be important in ensuring that those changes are contained when Congress negotiates the final budget bill.

Once a bill is passed and signed into law, it is assigned a session law number. The Balanced Budget Act of 1997 is also referred to as P.L. (for Public Law) 105-33.

Federal Regulations

Once a bill affecting the Medicare program becomes law, the responsibility for implementing and administering it falls to the Health Care Financing Administration (HCFA). HCFA is an agency within the U.S. Department of Health and Human Services that is responsible for administering the Medicare and Medicaid programs.

Like other federal agencies, one of the chief ways through which HCFA implements federal laws in its jurisdiction is by issuing federal regulations, also referred to as federal rules. Often, Congress will pass legislation that is general in nature and will leave it up to the implementing agency to provide the specifics. Sometimes legislation will be unclear (intentionally or not) about a specific aspect of how a law is to be carried out, or some confusion or disagreement about the details of a law will arise after it is passed.

Typically, HCFA will propose a new federal regulation, which will be published in the *Federal Register*, along with an explanation of the proposed regulation. After publication, interested members of the public have a period of time, generally 60 days, to offer comments. (Comments can support the proposal, oppose it, or suggest changes to be made before the proposal is finalized.) Sometime after the end of the comment period, HCFA issues the rules in final form, again published in the *Federal Register* along with an explanation of the changes made (if any), including a discussion of public comments received and an indication as to the effective date of the regulations. Sometimes HCFA will follow different procedures. For instance, it may issue an interim final rule, effective on or soon after publication, subject to change following public comment.

Needless to say, the "textbook" process for implementing federal rules is not always strictly followed-delays, sometimes lengthy (or seemingly permanent), often happen. For instance, HCFA never issued federal regulations implementing the NP and CNS reimbursement provisions of OBRA '90. Instead, it issued carrier instructions (described in the "Carrier Instructions" section) and left some of the details of implementing those provisions unclarified for several years. HCFA has issued regulations implementing the NP and CNS reimbursement provisions of the BBA, which were published in final form on November 2, 1998.

Once a rule takes effect, it is included in the *Code of Federal Regulations*, or CFR, which is a collection of federal rules issued by many federal agencies. Most of the federal rules relating to the Medicare and Medicaid programs can be found at Title 42 of the CFR.

Carrier Instructions

An important source for clarifying and implementing federal Medicare policy is through instructions issued to local Medicare contractors. As noted earlier, contractors responsible for implementing Medicare Part B are called Medicare carriers. HCFA issues carrier instructions to alert the carriers about new provisions in the law, new federal rules, and new procedures as well as to instruct them on HCFA's requirements for carrying out these provisions. Carrier instructions are collected in the *Medicare Carriers Manual*. Some important policies that do not appear in law or in the federal rules may be found in the *Carriers Manual*. For instance, HCFA's policies on payment for services provided incident to those of a physician are found in the *Medicare Carriers Manual* at Section 2050.

Carrier instructions can be issued more expeditiously than federal rules, so they have the advantage of allowing HCFA to move more quickly when time is an important consideration. (However, they do not allow for formal public input.) When the BBA was first enacted, for instance, HCFA issued carrier instructions in April 1998—four months after the effective date of the BBA provisions on NP and CNS reimbursement. These instructions informed carriers of the new law and told them to begin implementing it right away. This action meant that NPs and CNSs were able to obtain provider numbers and to submit claims for reimbursement without having to wait the additional seven months before final regulations were eventually issued.

Carrier Policies and Bulletins

Local Medicare carriers are responsible for administering the Medicare program in each state (or, in some cases, in part of a state). Carriers are given some discretion in administrative areas that are not addressed in Medicare law or rules or in HCFA instructions. However, carriers do not rewrite federal Medicare policy. When carriers misinterpret federal policy or adopt policies that conflict in some way with federal policy, HCFA can clarify and can help resolve the problem. For example, before the BBA when NP and CNS services were covered in rural areas only, some carriers were denying payment to NPs and CNSs who were billing for services provided in rural areas but whose office locations were located in non-rural areas. Although these carriers found it administratively convenient to accept or deny billing according to the practitioner's office location, the law provided for reimbursement based on where the service was provided. HCFA issued a memorandum to carriers clarifying the law and notifying them that eligible services provided in rural areas should be reimbursed regardless of the location of the NP's or CNS's office.

Other Sources

Other sources may have an effect, directly or indirectly, on Medicare law and policy. The federal courts are sometimes asked to rule on the constitutionality of federal laws or on whether specific federal regulations or policies are consistent with relevant Medicare statute, particularly in areas such as provision of the appeal rights of benefits and beneficiaries. State laws may also have an indirect effect on Medicare reimbursement for NPs and CNSs. As discussed in the section

"Legal Authorization to Perform Part B Services," services provided by NPs and CNSs must be within their scope of practice, which is defined by state law and regulations, to qualify for Medicare coverage. In addition, Medicare law and HCFA regulations require collaboration between NPs or CNSs and physicians that is, to a large extent, also a matter of state requirements. Thus, even though the Medicare program itself is an exclusively federal program, NPs and CNSs still need to be familiar with some aspects of state law to understand the services they can provide and the practice arrangements under which they must operate if they are to seek Medicare reimbursement.

MAKING SENSE OF MEDICARE COVERAGE OF NP AND CNS SERVICES

The Balanced Budget Act (BBA) of 1997 (P.L. 105-33) expanded the definition of physicians' services (i.e., reimbursable Part B services) to include the following:

… services which would be physicians' services if furnished by a physician … and which are performed by a nurse practitioner or clinical nurse specialist … working in collaboration with a physician … which the nurse practitioner or clinical nurse specialist is legally authorized to perform by the State in which the services are performed, and such services and supplies furnished as an incident to such services as would be covered … if furnished incident to a physician's professional services, but only if no facility or other provider charges or is paid any amounts with respect to the furnishing of such services. (BBA §4511)

This lengthy sentence includes a lot of information. It is probably most helpful to break it down into the specific issues it addresses or raises.

■ Who is considered a nurse practitioner (NP) or a clinical nurse specialist (CNS) under the law?

■ What does collaboration mean?

■ What does it mean to be legally authorized to perform services?

■ What does the language on "incident to" services mean?

■ What does the language about "only if no facility or other provider charges or is paid" mean?

Readers will recall that a number of sources of authority exists for Medicare law. Statute, as contained in legislation passed by Congress, is the starting point, but legislation is refined, clarified, and implemented by federal regulations (or rules) and often by policy memoranda issued by the relevant federal agency.

The 1997 law that provided for Medicare Part B coverage of NP and CNS services is a good example of this process. Passage of the law was followed by issuing a program memorandum and a set of rules to clarify and implement NP and CNS coverage. Understanding the new law means looking at all of these sources.

Questions and Answers on Current Medicare Law and Policy

Definitions of NP

The statute provides broad definitions of NP and CNS, which are made more specific by the regulations. The statute essentially provides that an NP is someone who is licensed as a registered nurse (RN) and who is authorized to practice as an NP and that a CNS is someone who is licensed as an RN and who holds a master's degree in a defined clinical area of nursing.

An early issue in implementing the law was the question of what level of education NPs must possess to qualify as Medicare providers. Initially, the Health Care Financing Administration (HCFA) proposed that all NPs must hold a master's degree. Although the American Nurses Association (ANA) and virtually all other nursing organizations agree that NPs should hold a master's degree or higher in nursing, most organizations were also concerned about an immediate requirement that NPs be prepared with a master's degree to bill Medicare for their services. Many NPs entered practice before master's degree-level NP programs were common. Imposing a requirement of a master's degree without any transition period would have excluded many experienced NPs from providing services to Medicare beneficiaries. Among those who could have been excluded were many NPs who were *already* providing Medicare services in rural areas under the Omnibus Budget Reconciliation Act of 1990 (OBRA '90). (HCFA had never required a master's degree for NPs providing services in rural areas under the old law.)

Although HCFA proposed a master's degree to bill Medicare, HCFA also proposed that NPs must be certified by a national certifying body. All of these bodies either currently require that applicants for certification hold a master's degree, or they are moving toward implementing such a requirement. But a great many NPs were certified before such requirements were in place.

Ultimately, HCFA adopted regulations that provide a transition to requiring a master's degree without excluding NPs currently in practice and who may lack this level of preparation.

1. An individual can qualify as an NP if she or he is an RN who is authorized to practice as an NP in the state in which services are provided *and* is certified by a recognized national certifying body that has established standards for NPs.

2. Alternatively, an individual can qualify as an NP if she or he is an RN who is authorized to practice by the state in which services are provided and she or he has been granted an NP provider number prior to December 31, 2000.

3. As of January 1, 2001, the alternative specified in (2) is no longer available. The individual must be authorized to practice in her or his state and must be certified by a recognized national certifying body that has established standards for NPs.

4. As of January 1, 2003, an NP who applies for a billing number for the first time must, in addition to the above, hold a master's degree in nursing.

These requirements allow for a transition to a master's degree requirement without excluding anyone who currently holds a billing number. It also provides enough advance notice so that NPs who are currently in practice and who lack a master's degree can apply for a billing number and so that NP students will know that they should seek master's degree preparation in nursing if they intend to bill Medicare for their services.

Prior to January 1, 2001	Must be an NP under your state's laws and *either* 1 be certified by a national body *or* 2 hold a Medicare provider number as of December 31, 2000
January 1, 2001 – January 1, 2003	Must be an NP under your state's laws *and* be certified by a national body
As of January 1, 2003	Must be an NP under your state's laws, be certified by a national body, *and* hold a master's degree in nursing

Note: The above dates indicate requirements for obtaining a billing number for the first time and for billing Medicare. Once an NP has obtained a Medicare number, she or he does not lose her or his status as an NP provider as requirements change.

Definition of CNS

A CNS must be an RN who is licensed and authorized to perform the services of a CNS in the state in which she or he practices, must hold a master's degree in a defined clinical area of nursing from an accredited educational institution, and must be certified by the American Nurses Credentialing Center (ANCC).

The issue of master's-level preparation has not proved to be a complicated one in determining qualifications for CNSs to bill Medicare. There are two reasons for this. First, master's degree preparation in nursing has been widely accepted as a requirement for CNS practice for some time. Second, the language of the statute explicitly requires that a CNS hold a master's degree.

Potentially less clear is the requirement that the CNS be an RN who is authorized to perform the services of a CNS in the state in which she or he practices. Some states explicitly recognize CNSs as a category of advanced practice registered nurse (APRN); many do not. The law does not require that a CNS practice in a state that explicitly recognizes CNSs, but rather that she or he be authorized to perform the services of a CNS. In many states, CNSs practice under the general authority of the state nurse practice act. In states that do require a specific mechanism or requirements for CNSs (such as state certification or title recognition), a CNS needs to meet those requirements in order to qualify for Medicare reimbursement.

Collaboration Requirement

The law requires that, in order to be covered by Medicare, services provided by an NP or a CNS must be performed in collaboration with a physician. State laws vary widely as to what kind of relationship they require between NPs and physicians or between CNSs and physicians. Many states have no specific requirements for collaboration with physicians, leaving practice arrangements up to individual NPs, CNSs, and physicians.

In implementing the law's requirement for collaboration, Medicare regulations define collaboration as a process in which an NP or CNS works with one or more physicians to deliver health care services within the scope of the practitioner's expertise, with medical direction and appropriate supervision as provided for in jointly developed guidelines or other mechanisms as provided by the law of the state in which the services are performed (42 CFR 410.75 and 410.76).

The regulations also recognize that some states have no specific requirement for collaboration or do not mandate the details of a collaborative relationship. Thus, the regulations go on to explain that in the absence of state law governing collaboration, collaboration is a process in which an NP or CNS has a relationship with one or more physicians to deliver health care services. Such collaboration is to be evidenced by NPs or CNSs documenting their scope of practice and by indicating the relationships they have with physicians to deal with issues outside their scope of practice. NPs and CNSs must document this collaborative relationship with physicians. The regulations also explain that the collaborating physician does not need to be present with the NP or CNS when services are delivered nor does the physician need to make an independent evaluation of each patient who is seen by the NP or CNS.

It should be emphasized that the collaboration requirement must be met if services furnished by an NP or CNS are to qualify for Medicare reimbursement, even if an NP or CNS is practicing in a state that has no legal requirements whatsoever for collaboration. In other words, for those NPs and CNSs, requirements that must be met for services to qualify for Medicare reimbursement may go beyond the requirements they must meet to practice. The regulations do, however, recognize that some states do not require collaboration and have provided for less restrictive collaboration requirements to apply in those states.

Legal Authorization to Perform Part B Services

The law requires that, to qualify for Medicare coverage, services performed by an NP or a CNS be services that the NP or CNS is legally authorized to perform. This requirement means that the services the NP or CNS is providing must be within her or his legal scope of practice. In most states, the scope of practice for APRNs is determined by the state nursing practice act and by state board of nursing rules and policies. (In some states, the state medical board may also have a role in regulating advanced nursing practice and may have a say in determining scope of practice). The basic idea is that if an NP or a CNS is performing a service that she or he is not legally authorized to perform, Medicare will not pay for it.

Incident to Services

As we have already discussed in the section "Direct and Indirect Medicare Payment," for many years the only way that services provided by NPs or CNSs could be covered by Medicare was under the "incident to" provision (i.e., the part of Medicare law that provides for coverage of services and supplies furnished incident to the professional services of a physician). The same arrangements that apply to services provided incident to those of a physician apply to services provided incident to those of an NP or a CNS. *Medicare Carriers Manual* Section 2050 spells out the requirements for services provided incident to those of a physician. The requirements for services provided incident to those of an NP or a CNS are spelled out in the federal regulations (42 CFR Sections 410.75(d) and 410.76(d)). The service may be covered if

- It would be covered if furnished by a physician or as incident to the professional services of a physician,

- It is of the type commonly furnished in a physician's office and either furnished without charge or included in the bill for the NP's or CNS's service,

- It is an incidental but integral part of the professional service performed by the NP or the CNS, and

- It is performed under the direct supervision of the NP or CNS (she or he must be physically present and immediately available).

Some of the details of payment for services provided incident to those of a physician are instructive in determining when services provided incident to those of an NP or a CNS may be covered. For instance, services provided incident to those of a physician generally must be provided by an employee of the physician or by an individual who shares a common employer with the physician (for instance, if an NP and physician are both employed by the same community clinic.)

A similar relationship is most likely contemplated by the regulations; in other words, the services be delivered by an individual (e.g., a staff nurse, medical assistant, or other office staff member) who is employed by the NP or CNS or who shares a common employer. The requirement for physical presence and immediate availability have been interpreted to mean (as regards "incident to" payments to physicians) that the physician must be present in the same office suite where services are delivered; it appears likely that the same interpretation would apply to services provided incident to those of an NP or a CNS. In other words, the NP or CNS be present in the same office suite where services are provided by a staff nurse or other office staff member.

No Dual Payment

The law provides that payment for NP and CNS services can be made when appropriate requirements are met, "but only if no facility or other provider charges or is paid any amounts with respect to the furnishing of such services." The regulations repeat this exclusion (42 CFR Sections 410.75(e), 410.76(e)).

Essentially, this statement means that Medicare will not pay twice for the same service. Some of the kinds of payment that could be excluded by this provision may seem a matter of common sense. For instance, if a physician has billed for services provided by an NP as services furnished incident to the physician's professional services, the NP cannot then bill Medicare for the same services.

The memorandum issued by HCFA in April 1998 and the regulations issued in November 1998 address this exclusion in part. When services of NPs or CNSs are bundled into a capitated Part B payment, Medicare will not separately pay for NP or CNS services, because these services are paid for as part of the bundled payment. However, the settings in which Part B payments are bundled into capitated payment are rare; thus, HCFA indicates that the only settings in which separate payment are categorically excluded are in rural health clinics and federally qualified health centers.

Although no other settings are categorically excluded, it is likely that questions will arise over payment for NP and CNS services in other settings.

One area that remains to be fully clarified is billing for services provided to hospital inpatients. It appears clear that NPs and CNSs who are not employees of the hospital (i.e., those professionals who are in their own practices or who are in physician practices) should be able to bill (or the practice should be able to bill) for hospital visits. However, some NPs and CNSs have raised concerns as to whether such services can be billed when they are provided by hospital employees. This situation has been a source of confusion for many, including NPs, CNSs, and carriers. Again, ANA is working to achieve clarification of some of the questions involved, but no resolution has yet been achieved.

The authors believe that a fair reading of the law would be that services provided by NPs and CNSs to hospital inpatients can be covered by Medicare Part B as long as they are otherwise eligible for reimbursement (e.g., if the services would be covered if provided by a physician, are within the scope of practice of the NP or CNS, and meet the other requirements contained in the law and regulations). The employment status of the NP or CNS should not be a determinative factor. Some have suggested that because hospital-employed NPs and CNSs receive their salaries from the hospital, these salary costs are paid for by Medicare Part A, and, therefore, their services must be excluded from Part B coverage because the facility "charges or is paid … for the furnishing of" these services.

However, this is not necessarily the case. Nursing services are included in the diagnosis-related group (DRG) payment that the hospital receives for each patient under the Medicare prospective payment system (PPS). The hospital receives a bundled, prospectively determined payment amount for each inpatient. Although it includes nursing services, it does not include professional services (i.e., physicians' services), which are generally covered under Part B. Prior to the passage of the BBA, physicians' services provided by NPs and CNSs were essentially unpaid by Medicare: They are not reflected in the Part A payment and were not eligible for payment under Part B.

The type of service determines whether an NP or CNS service can be paid by Part B. Hospital visits and other physicians' services should be eligible for coverage. Services that are more like routine inpatient nursing services or that are adjunct to or that support those services (consultation to nursing staff, serving as a clinical resource, conducting education or support activities for nursing staff) *are* arguably included in the Part A payment and probably could not be paid under Part B. (They are also generally not of a type that would qualify for Part B payment anyway.)

Many hospitals employ physicians on staff to provide professional services to hospitalized patients, and their services generally qualify for Part B coverage. The authors believe that a strong case exists for treating services of hospital-employed NPs and CNSs in the same manner that services of hospital-employed attending physicians are treated. The fact that NPs and CNSs are nurses does not mean that they are providers of inpatient nursing services reflected in the DRG payment.

Resolution of these issues will involve continued discussions with HCFA, local carriers, and hospital administrators.

Other Reimbursement Issues

Payment Amount

Medicare will pay an NP or a CNS 80 percent of the lesser of the actual charge or 85 percent of the amount that is paid to physicians under the Medicare Fee Schedule. In essence, this statement means that NPs and CNSs are paid 85 percent of what physicians are paid for a given service. Medicare payment is always based on the lesser of the fee schedule amount or the amount actually charged. An NP, CNS, or physician can choose to charge a lower amount than he or she is legally entitled to; in such a case, Medicare will only pay the amount charged, not the full fee schedule amount. In addition, readers should recall that Medicare generally pays only 80 percent of charges for physicians' services; beneficiaries are responsible for a 20 percent co-payment.

Medicare law provides that services provided by an NP or a CNS are discounted; that is, they are paid at 85 percent of what a physician is paid. Thus, if the allowable charge for a given service is $100, Medicare would pay a physician $80; the beneficiary would be responsible for $20. If an NP or CNS performs the service, the total allowable charge is $85. Medicare will pay the NP or CNS $68 (85 percent of $80), and the beneficiary will be responsible for $17 (20 percent of $80).

Accepting Assignment

Medicare law requires that NPs and CNSs accept assignment. This requirement means that the NPs and CNSs agree to accept the Medicare Fee Schedule amount as payment in full and cannot bill a patient for any amount beyond that. This requirement does *not* mean that the NP or CNS cannot collect the 20 percent co-payment from the patient (the remaining $17 in the example given above). It *does* mean that the NP or CNS cannot decide that she or he wants to charge an amount above the Medicare Fee Schedule and collect on that higher amount.

Professional Services

For an NP or a CNS to charge Medicare for services, the services must be provided directly by the NP or CNS, or alternatively the services may qualify as services provided "incident to" those of an NP or CNS. Merely supervising other staff members does not constitute personal performance of a professional service by an NP or a CNS.

Mental Health Services

Generally, the law does not make a distinction among those professional services that Medicare will pay for when provided by an NP or a CNS. Under most circumstances, if a physician can be paid for it, so can an NP or a CNS, as long as all other requirements are met (such as being authorized by state law to perform the service and performing the service in collaboration with a physician).

However, during the initial months of implementing Medicare reimbursement for NPs and CNSs, some concerns arose as to whether or not NPs and CNSs could be reimbursed for mental health services. Those concerns are addressed in the text preceding the HCFA final rule on NP and CNS reimbursement, which was published in the November 2, 1998, *Federal Register*. (The text preceding a federal rule is commonly called the *preamble*.) Although the preamble does not generally appear in the regulations themselves, it carries important weight because it explains the thinking of the federal agency responsible for issuing and implementing the regulations (in this case, HCFA).

On the issue of mental health services provided by NPs and CNSs, HCFA explains

… it is our understanding that some nurse practitioners and clinical nurse specialists specialize in mental health. Therefore, if State law authorizes these nonphysician practitioners to perform mental health services and evaluation and management services that would otherwise be furnished by a physician … psychiatric nurse practitioners and clinical nurse specialists could bill for psychiatric diagnostic interviews and any of the psychotherapy CPT codes that include medical evaluation and management. (HCFA 1998)

Ordering Tests and Services

The question of whether and when NPs and CNSs can order diagnostic tests or specific types of services is separate from the question of which services NPs and CNSs themselves can provide. An NP or a CNS may be able to provide (and be paid for) a range of health care services; but if Medicare will not recognize her or his ability to order laboratory tests or physical therapy services (both of which would be provided by someone else), then her or his ability to provide primary or specialty care may be significantly compromised. Medicare regulations address some of these concerns.

Medicare rules generally require that diagnostic x-ray tests, laboratory tests, and other diagnostic tests be ordered by the physician who is treating the patient. Tests not ordered by the treating physician are "not reasonable and necessary"; that is, Medicare will not pay for them (42 CFR 410.32(a)). NPs and CNSs who "furnish services that would be physician services if furnished by a physician, and who are operating within their authority under State law and within the scope of their Medicare statutory benefit, may be treated the same as physicians treating beneficiaries for the purposes of" this rule (*ibid.*). In other words, NPs and CNSs may order diagnostic tests as part of providing professional services to a patient, as long as those services are within their scope of practice and otherwise qualify for Medicare payment (42 CFR 410.32(a)(3)). Moreover, Medicare will pay for diagnostic tests performed by NPs or CNSs if they are authorized to perform them under state law (42 CFR 410.32(b)(2)(v)).

Medicare will pay for physical therapy, occupational therapy, and speech-language pathology services when these services have been ordered by NPs and CNSs, as long as these services are medically reasonable and necessary and state law authorizes them to do so. NPs and CNSs can also certify and recertify the plan of treatment for these services if they are authorized to do so (42 CFR Sections 410.60, 410.61, and 410.62).

MEDICARE BILLING BASICS

Enrolling as a Medicare Provider

Enrolling as a Medicare Part B provider gives you the opportunity to bill Medicare directly for the services you provide as an advanced practice registered nurse (APRN). It also guarantees that the services you provide will be included in the Medicare database so that Medicare data accurately reflect the extent and level of services that APRNs provide to Medicare beneficiaries.

Becoming a participating Part B provider involves the following process.

1. Start by creating a file of documents you will need to have available at your practice site. These include: your state authorization to practice as an APRN (license and/or state certification), your scope of practice as defined in state statute or in state rules or regulations, your professional malpractice insurance policy, and documentation of your collaborative agreement with a physician or physicians for consultation and referrals. If your state statute or regulations include a definition of the APRN–physician collaborative agreement, your agreement must meet any requirements in that definition. If your state does not include a definition, then your collaborative agreement must meet the requirements of collaboration as defined in CFR Section 410.75 (Appendix A. 1).

2. Contact the Professional Relations Department of the Medicare Part B Carrier for your region and request a provider enrollment application to become a Medicare provider. If you do not know the Medicare Part B Carrier for your region, the list of Medicare carriers with addresses and phone numbers is available on the Health Care Financing Administration (HCFA) Website at <www/ hcfa.gov/medicare/incardir.htm#1>.

3. Fill out the health care provider application form (HCFA 855) for initial enrollment in the program. Follow the detailed instructions included with the form (Appendix B. 1 and Appendix C. 1) to fill out the application accurately and completely. It is often helpful to work with your practice business manager to complete the application successfully.

Group Practice

For Medicare billing purposes, a group practice is defined as a partnership, association, or corporation composed of two or more physicians, nonphysician practitioners, or both who wish to bill Medicare as a unit. If you choose to file claims as part of a group practice, the entire group must request a group provider number and bill using that number. Each member within the group must also be enrolled in the Medicare program as an individual to enroll as a member of a group. In addition, each member within the group must complete a reassignment of benefits form (HCFA Form 855R; Appendix B. 5), stating that she or he agrees to turn the money over to the group that Medicare would normally pay each of them directly. After the agreement has been signed, your Medicare carrier may assign each individual provider Medicare number a unique identifier that must be submitted when billing.

Medicare Provider Identification

Changes in provider information, such as your name, practice site, or specialty, must be reported to the Medicare program on the HCFA Form 855C (Appendix B. 3).

To bill Medicare directly, you must have a provider identification number (PIN). When your Medicare enrollment form is completed and approved, the Medicare carrier in your region will issue you a PIN to be used when billing Medicare for the services you deliver to Medicare beneficiaries. PINs can be either numeric, alphanumeric, or all alpha, depending on your regional carrier. The PIN number will automatically be deactivated if it is not used for 12 consecutive months. A new HCFA Form 855 must be completed and approved to reactivate the billing number. In the future, PINs will be replaced nationally by a national provider identification (NPI) number that will stay with you as a Medicare provider throughout your affiliation with the Medicare program in any state in which you provide Medicare Part B services.

In addition to your PIN, you will also be issued a unique provider identification number (UPIN) to use on the HCFA 1500 claim form in block 17 and 17(a) whenever you are ordering or referring services for Medicare beneficiaries. Prior to January 1, 1999, nurse practitioners (NPs), clinical nurse specialists (CNSs), and physicians assistants (PAs) were required to use a surrogate UPIN, NPP000, because individual UPINs had not been issued to them. However, because individual UPINs are now issued at enrollment, the surrogate UPIN NPP00 is no longer to be used. Claims containing the surrogate UPIN will be returned as unprocessable (Appendix C. 3).

When you have obtained your PIN from the regional Medicare Part B Carrier, you can start to bill Medicare by documenting your services according to the allowable charges by using the Medicare Part B Physician Fee Schedule. Remember your PIN should be protected just as a credit card number should, because it is your personal identifier within the Medicare program. For your own protection against any fraud and abuse charges, you need to make sure that no one uses your PIN to bill Medicare without your authorization. Most important, remember that providers are responsible for all the claims submitted and billed on their behalf.

Additional identifying letters or numbers known as modifiers are no longer required on Medicare claims submitted by NPs and CNSs. This policy change became effective April 1, 1999. Claims must be reported by using the PIN, and payment for claims will be based on the PIN. However, there is one exception to this policy: A modifier (AS-) will continue to be used when billing for services provided by NPs or CNSs when they are performing as assistants-at-surgery (Appendix C. 3).

Medicare Payment Methodology

Agreeing to participate as a Medicare provider means that you agree to accept Medicare's allowable charge as payment in full for the Part B services that you provide. Medicare will determine the allowable charge then reimburses you as an NP/CNS at 85 percent of the amount that a physician would receive as a reimbursable charge. The remaining 20 percent coinsurance is the patient's responsibility. Medicare requires that beneficiaries pay coinsurance for most services. Providing the service at no charge to the beneficiary and billing Medicare for that service constitutes a routine waiver of coinsurance and is considered unlawful.

The Medicare payment methodology and rates for certified registered nurse anesthetists (CRNAs) and certified nurse-midwives (CNMs) are each different and have been determined by statute, regulation, or both. See Appendix A. 6, 7, and 8.

Opting Out of the Medicare Program

Section 4507 of the Balanced Budget Act (BBA) of 1997 (P.L. 150-33) permits physicians and practitioners to *opt out* of the Medicare program and enter into private contracts with Medicare beneficiaries, if specific requirements are met. When you opt out, none of the services provided by you are covered by Medicare, and no Medicare payments will be made to you directly or on a capitated basis. Additionally, no Medicare payment may be made to the beneficiary for your services if you have opted out of the program. Under the statute, you cannot choose to opt out for some Medicare beneficiaries but not for others.

To enter into a private contract with a beneficiary, you must opt out of Medicare and file an affidavit with your Medicare carrier, advising that you have opted out of Medicare. The affidavit must be filed within 10 days of entering into the first private contract with a Medicare beneficiary and must state that you will not submit any claim to Medicare for any item or service provided to any Medicare beneficiary during the two-year period beginning on the date the affidavit is filed.

In a private contract, the Medicare beneficiary agrees to give up Medicare payment for services furnished by the opted out provider and to pay the provider without regard to any limits that would otherwise apply to what the provider could charge.

When a provider, who has opted out of the Medicare program, provides emergency care to a Medicare beneficiary, then a modifier (GJ) is appended to the service code to designate opt-out physician or practitioner emergency or urgent services. The use of the modifier (GJ) on the claim form indicates that the service was provided by an opt-out physician or practitioner who has not signed a private contract with the Medicare beneficiary for emergency or urgent care furnished to the beneficiary.

Medicare Managed Care

If you plan to provide Medicare Part B services to a Medicare beneficiary who is enrolled in a Medicare managed care plan, you will have to apply to the managed care plan for admission to the plan's panel or list of primary care providers. When Medicare beneficiaries enroll in a managed care plan, they select a primary care provider from the plan's list of primary care providers, and the primary care provider becomes responsible for coordinating all of their health care services. HCFA contracts with managed care plans to provide Medicare benefits and reimburses the plans according to an adjusted capitation rate that is paid on a monthly basis. Each managed care plan has its own network of hospitals, skilled nursing facilities, home health agencies, and health care professionals who provide the Medicare services according to the terms or conditions of negotiated contracts between the providers and the plan.

To become a member of a managed care plan's panel of providers, start by contacting the provider relations department of the managed care plan to request an application for admission to the panel of providers. Fill out the application completely and accurately and return it. If you are offered admission to the panel as a primary care provider, you will be offered a contract with the managed care plan. However, before you sign a contract with a managed care plan, it is advisable to seek legal counsel to review the terms of the contract, as it will typically cover many other issues concerning your practice, as well as how you are reimbursed for your services.

If your application is denied, you will want to follow up and find out the reason for rejection. There may be actions you can take to challenge or change the initial denial. Being admitted to a managed care plan's panel of primary care providers still takes patience and persistence in many regions of the country. Barriers to inclusion on managed care panels and arbitrary restrictions to APRN practice included in managed care contracts, such as adding physician supervision requirements, adding needless patient record cosignatory requirements, or restricting prescription privileges, still exist and adversely affect managed care reimbursement and utilization of APRNs.

Billing for Medicare Services Using the Medicare Part B Fee Schedule

Payment for Medicare Part B services is based on a Medicare Physician Fee Schedule that is updated annually by HCFA. The fee schedule is based on a resource-based relative value system (RBRVS), using a complex formula that establishes a fee for each service or procedure code. The formula includes three components: the professional work required for the service or procedure, which takes into consideration the time, intensity, and technical skill required to provide the service; the practice expenses, such as office staff salaries, supplies, equipment, rent; and the professional liability insurance premium associated with the service or procedure. The relative value for these three components is then adjusted, using three geographical cost indexes (GCIs) and then multiplied by a national conversion factor to arrive at a the geographic-specific fee schedule for a particular area for each procedure or service code, setting the reimbursement rate for the providers of that particular procedure or service. The relative unit values (RUVs), GCIs, and conversion factor are updated annually with implementation beginning on January 1 of each year. The revisions are printed in the *Federal Register* in November of the previous year. The Medicare Fee Schedule conversion factor for the year 2000 is $36.6137.

Submitting Claims to Medicare

Providers must submit professional service claims for Medicare beneficiaries on the HCFA 1500 form or by electronic media claims (EMC) transmission. The proper, accurate, and timely completion and submission of a claim is the first step to ensure that your claim will be processed as expediently as possible.

Detailed guidelines for completing a HCFA 1500 claim form are available through your regional Medicare Part B Carrier (Appendix B. 3). It is the responsibility of the health care professional to accurately report the level or type of service provided to patients according to the coding guidelines and HCFA rules. To receive prompt payment, you must fully and accurately complete a total of 33 items on the HCFA 1500 form.

As a participating Medicare provider, you can become familiar with the billing and coding process by referring to billing and coding resource materials that are widely available. (See Bibliography.) The Medicare Carriers also issue Medicare Part B Bulletins with the latest coding changes and implementation dates to keep you updated on reimbursement policy and procedures. Learning to use the codes appropriately to document and to report your services will help ensure proper payment and will help reduce the likelihood of a Medicare audit of your practice.

EMC is a claims submission process that transmits Medicare Part B claims electronically by modem from your office computer to the Medicare Part B carrier for immediate claims processing, 24 hours a day, 7 days a week. EMC filing is quicker and payment is released as soon as HCFA time-frame requirements for claims payments have been satisfied. Payment for electronic claims is made 14 days after the date of receiving the claim as opposed to 27 days for paper claims. Once the claim is received, it is electronically checked for the correct information. Claims that pass these initial checks are either processed and paid if the service is allowed by Medicare Part B or sent back, usually for additional information. The business manager at your practice site is the key resource for more information on the EMC mode of claims submission.

Coding Procedures

All Medicare carriers process claims by using the American Medical Association coding system, the Current Procedural Terminology (CPT), and the Health Care Financing Administration's Common Procedure Coding System (HCPCS). Each procedure you perform and charge to Medicare must have either a CPT or HCPCS code to describe what service was provided.

The CPT is a listing of more than 7,000 codes used to report procedures and services that providers perform. The CPT code communicates to Medicare what you did when you saw the patient. CPT codes are five-digit numbers with narrative descriptions that provide a uniform language that serves as an effective means of communication among providers, patients, and third-party payers. All third-party payers accept CPT codes, including managed care organizations. Procedures are grouped within six major sections: evaluation and management (E&M), anesthesiology, surgery, radiology, pathology and laboratory, and medicine. Within each section are subsections with anatomic, procedural, condition, or descriptor subheadings. *Physicians' Current Procedural Terminology CPT 2000*, a complete list of all current CPT codes, is available for purchase from the American Medical Association (AMA).

HCPCS (pronounced hick-picks) is a three-level coding system developed by HCFA for documenting Part B Medicare services. Level I is the CPT code. Level II is a national alphanumeric code that begins with a letter followed by four numbers used primarily to report supplies and injections to Medicare and other payers. Level III is a state alphanumeric code and contains codes assigned and maintained by individual state carriers. Individual carriers assign these codes to describe new procedures that are not yet available in Level I or Level II codes.

In addition to CPT and HCPCS codes, it is also necessary to provide Medicare with the correct patient diagnosis coded to the highest level of specificity. A diagnosis is identified on the claim form by using the *International Classification of Diseases*, Ninth Revision, Clinical Modification (ICD-9-CM). This identification is a three- to five-digit numeric or alphanumeric code that describes the patient's diagnosis or symptoms and justifies why a test or service was ordered or provided to the patient.

CPT and HCPCS code modifiers are used to provide additional information to the payer and, in some circumstances, will affect the reimbursement rate. Modifiers indicate that a service or procedure has been altered by some specific circumstance but that its definition or code has not changed.

Reimbursement Exceptions

Medicare will not reimburse for the following three categories of services: (1) services that Medicare never pays for (basically noncovered services); (2) services that are included or bundled in the payment for another service; and (3) services considered not to be medically necessary.

Some of the noncovered services include routine annual physicals; acupuncture; screening tests with no documented conditions or symptoms; routine foot care; cosmetic surgery; personal convenience items; examinations for the purpose of prescribing eye glasses or hearing aid; and services, drugs, and devices not considered safe and effective because they are experimental or investigational.

If another facility or provider charges or is paid any amount for the Part B services you have provided, Medicare payment to you will be denied. HCFA will not pay twice for the same service. For example, Medicare payments are made to rural health centers and federally qualified health centers under an all-inclusive rate that specifically accounts for the services of health professionals working in these settings because the facility payment rate reflects the costs for these services. If you are employed at a rural health center or federally qualified health center, you are not permitted to bill Medicare directly for your services because your payment is bundled into the facility payment rate.

Medicare will not pay for services that are not reasonable and necessary for the diagnosis or for the treatment of an illness or injury. A service may also be considered not reasonable and necessary if the frequency or duration of the service was provided beyond the accepted standards of professional practice. Claims for these services will be denied. Providers who do not want to assume financial responsibility for the denied service should give the patient an acceptable advanced notice of Medicare's denial or reduction of payment. The patient can then decide if he or she wants the service and is willing to pay for it. Ask the patient to sign a waiver of liability statement before the service is provided that indicates a description of the procedure or service, the specific reason that you think it will not be covered, and the estimated cost of payment. On the HCFA 1500 claim form, the modifier -GA must be appended to the procedure code to indicate that the waiver of liability statement is on file.

Documentation of Evaluation and Management Services

E&M service codes are the most frequently used codes by APRNs. For E&M services, the nature and amount of professional work and documentation varies by type of service, place of service, and the patient's status. The descriptors for the levels of E&M services recognize seven components that are used in defining levels of E&M services. These components include the following:

- History

- Examination

- Nature of presenting problem

- Medical decision making

- Counseling

- Coordination of care

- Time

All providers who are authorized to provide E&M services use the same CPT codes for reporting their services regardless of specialty. For this system to work, all providers must use E&M codes that are based on a consistent understanding of the coding and documentation criteria. In 1995, HCFA, working with the American Medical Association and a number of professional organizations, developed a set of E&M coding guidelines which were designed to help providers increase accuracy and to improve consistency when reporting E&M services. The guidelines are considered instructional material that represent HCFA policy regarding interpretation of E&M codes and the medical documentation required to support a recorded level of code. In 1997, the E&M guidelines were rewritten to define with greater clinical specificity the content of the general multi-system examinations, the documentation requirements for general multi-system examinations were revised, and definitions for organ-specific or body system-specific examinations were added. Many providers expressed concerns that the 1997 guidelines were too cumbersome to use in practice and that their use could detract from patient care. Additional attempts to respond to these provider concerns resulted in the development of an alternative set of guidelines that are based on the 1995 guidelines. These alternative guidelines (referred to by HCFA as "June 2000 Documentation

Guidelines") are being pilot tested before they are implemented. During the pilot study period, and until new guidelines are finally implemented, Medicare carriers have been instructed to continue review of medical records according to the 1995 or 1997 documentation guidelines. Currently, providers may use either 1995 or 1997 guidelines to document E&M services, whichever is most advantageous to the provider. The 1995 and the 1997 Evaluation and Management Guidelines are included in Appendix D.

Claim Denials

A number of ways exist to appeal Medicare decisions. Your regional Medicare Carrier Provider Customer Service can provide you with information about your Medicare claims and can provide key explanations about why your claim was denied. Certain types of claim denials can generally be handled by a telephone review request. Your carrier will provide you with information about telephone review. If a charge can be submitted as either a new claim or a telephone review, Medicare generally encourages refiling your claim because this is normally the most efficient way to receive payment.

Once your review request is processed, you will receive a written response, notifying you of the carrier's decision. In any review letter, you will be advised of your rights to a Medicare Part B hearing, should you choose to request one. Hearings are conducted by a Medicare-appointed hearing officer whose role is to determine whether the carrier has followed Medicare guidelines in making the determination in question. A request for a hearing must be filed within six months from the date of the denial notification.

The three types of hearings are as follows:

1. On-the-record decisions. This type is the easiest and most convenient hearing. You can request in writing for a hearing or submit a Fair Hearing HCFA 1965 form. A decision can be made quickly on the basis of the facts in the file and any additional information you send to the hearing officer.

2. Telephone hearing. This type of hearing offers a less costly alternative to the in-person hearing because the need to appear is eliminated. Oral testimony and oral challenge may be conducted by phone.

3. In-person hearing. As a provider, you are given the opportunity to present oral testimony supporting your claim and refuting or challenging the information the carrier used to deny your claim. This approach is more costly and time consuming.

The decision made by the hearing officer in many cases is final and binding. However, if more than $500 remains in controversy following the decision by the hearing officer, further consideration may be made by an Administrative Law Judge.

Fraud and Abuse

The issue of fraud and abuse has been prominent in discussions about how to improve the financial health of the Medicare program. Recent legislative action and other HCFA initiatives to combat fraud and abuse contain significant new antifraud and abuse provisions that increase penalties and have provided added financial resources for fighting fraud and abuse in the Medicare program. As a participating Medicare provider, your challenge is to practice, document, and bill for your services in compliance with a number of laws, regulations, and Medicare program requirements.

HCFA defines fraud as the intentional deception or misrepresentation that a person knows to be false or does not believe to be true and makes, knowing that the deception could result in some unauthorized benefit to himself or herself or to some other person. The most frequent kind of fraud arises from a false statement or from misrepresentation made or caused to be made that is related to entitlement or payment under the Medicare program. The violator may be a physician or other practitioner, a hospital or other institutional provider, a clinical laboratory or other supplier, an employee of any provider, a billing service, a beneficiary, Medicare carrier employee, or any other person in a position to bill the Medicare program.

Abuse involves the payment for items or services when no legal entitlement exists to that payment and the provider has not knowingly or intentionally misrepresented the facts to obtain payment. Abuse of the program may result in unnecessary costs to the Medicare program, improper payment, or payment for services that do not meet the professionally recognized standards of care.

In the Medicare program, the most common examples of fraud, abuse, or both include the following:

- Billing for services not furnished

- Misrepresenting the diagnosis to justify payment

- Billing for services as if they were performed by you when they were performed by a non-eligible Medicare provider

- Routinely waiving the coinsurance requirement for Medicare beneficiaries

- Misrepresenting as medically necessary services by using inappropriate procedure or diagnostic codes

- Billing for services in excess of those needed by the patient

When HCFA determines that fraud and abuse of the Medicare program potentially exists, the case is developed through research and investigation, then it is referred to the Office of the Inspector General. When discovered, fraudulent and abusive practices are dealt with by a wide range of enforcement actions, including application of administrative sanctions, such as exclusion from Medicare participation, civil and criminal monetary penalties, and criminal prosecution.

References

American Medical Association. 1999. *International classification of diseases.* 9th Revision, clinical modification (ICD-9-CM). 2 vols. Chicago: American Medical Association.

Balanced Budget Act of 1997. U.S. Public Law 105-33. 1 January 1998.

42 CFR 410.32(a)(3) (1999).

42 CFR 410.32(b)(2)(v) (1999).

42 CFR Sections 410.75(d) and 410.76(d) (1999).

42 CFR Sections 410.75(e) and 410.76(e) (1999).

42 CFR Sections 410.60, 410.61, and 410.62 (1998).

42 CFR 410.75 and 410.76 (1998).

Health Care Financing Administration (HCFA). 1998. Medicare program; revisions to payment policies and adjustments to the relative value units under the physician fee schedule for calendar year 1999: final rule. *Federal Register* 63, no. 211 (2 November): 59380–590.

———. Section 2050. *Medicare carriers manual.* Rockville, Maryland: U.S. Department of Health and Human Services, Health Care Financing Administration.

Mittelstadt, P., ed. 1993. *The reimbursement manual: How to get paid for your advanced practice nursing services.* Washington, D.C.: American Nurses Association.

Bibliography

American Medical Association. 2000. *Physicians' current procedural terminology*. CPT professional edition. Chicago: American Medical Association.

———. 1999. *HCPCS 2000 Medicare's national level II codes*. Chicago: American Medical Association.

———. 1999. *Principles of CPT coding*. Chicago: American Medical Association.

Blue Cross Blue Shield of Florida, Inc. et al. 1998. *Medicare fraud and abuse: A practical guide of proactive measures to avoid becoming a victim*. Jacksonville: Blue Cross Blue Shield of Florida.

Buppert, C.. 2000. *The primary care provider's guide to compensation and quality: How to get paid and not get sued*. Gaithersburg, Maryland: Aspen Publishers.

———. 1999. *Nurse practitioner's business practice and legal guide*. Gaithersburg, Maryland: Aspen Publishers.

Medical Learning Inc. 2000. *Nurse practitioner's guide to evaluation and management coding*. St. Paul, Minnesota: Medical Learning Inc.

Health Care Financing Administration (HCFA). 1999. Medicare program; revisions to payment policies under the physician fee schedule for calendar year 2000: final rule. 1999. *Federal Register* 64, 211 (2 November): 59380–590.

———. 1998. Medicare program; revisions to payment policies and adjustments to the relative value units under the physician fee schedule for calendar year 1999: final rule. *Federal Register* 63, 211 (2 November): 58814–914.

Richmond, T. H. Thompson, and E. Sullivan-Marx. 2000. Reimbursement for acute care nurse practitioner services. *American Journal of Critical Care* 9, 1:52–61.

Appendix A

Selected Sections of the Code of Federal Regulations

Appendix A.1

42 CFR §410.75
Nurse practitioners' services.

(a) *Definition.* As used in this section, the term "physician" means a doctor of medicine or osteopathy, as set forth in section [1861(r)(1)] 1861(r)(1)of the Act.

(b) *Qualifications.* For Medicare Part B coverage of his or her services, a nurse practitioner must—

    (1)   (i) Be a registered professional nurse who is authorized by the State in which the services are furnished to practice as a nurse practitioner in accordance with State law; and

        (ii) Be certified as a nurse practitioner by a recognized national certifying body that has established standards for nurse practitioners; or

    (2) Be a registered professional nurse who is authorized by the State in which the services are furnished to practice as a nurse practitioner in accordance with State law and have been granted a Medicare billing number as a nurse practitioner by December 31, 2000; or

    (3) Be a nurse practitioner who on or after January 1, 2001, applies for a Medicare billing number for the first time and meets the standards for nurse practitioners in paragraphs [42 CFR 410.75(b)(1)(i)] (b)(1)(i) and [42 CFR 410.75(b)(1)(ii)] (b)(1)(ii) of this section; or

    (4) Be a nurse practitioner who on or after January 1, 2003, applies for a Medicare billing number for the first time and possesses a master's degree in nursing and meets the standards for nurse practitioners in paragraphs [42 CFR 410.75(b)(1)(i)] (b)(1)(i) and [42 CFR 410.75(b)(1)(ii)] (b)(1)(ii) of this section.

(c) *Services.* Medicare Part B covers nurse practitioners' services in all settings in both rural and urban areas, only if the services would be covered if furnished by a physician and the nurse practitioner—

    (1) Is legally authorized to perform them in the State in which they are performed;

    (2) Is not performing services that are otherwise excluded from coverage because of one of the statutory exclusions; and

    (3) Performs them while working in collaboration with a physician.

        (i) Collaboration is a process in which a nurse practitioner works with one or more physicians to deliver health care services within the scope of the practitioner's expertise, with medical direction and appropriate supervision as provided for in jointly developed guidelines or other mechanisms as provided by the law of the State in which the services are performed.

        (ii) In the absence of State law governing collaboration, collaboration is a process in which a nurse practitioner has a relationship with one or more physicians to deliver health care services. Such collaboration is to be evidenced by nurse practitioners documenting the nurse practitioners' scope of practice and indicating the relationships that they have with physicians to deal with issues outside their scope of practice. Nurse practitioners must document this collaborative process with physicians.

(iii)   The collaborating physician does not need to be present with the nurse practitioner when the services are furnished or to make an independent evaluation of each patient who is seen by the nurse practitioner.

(d)   *Services and supplies incident to a nurse practitioners' services.* Medicare Part B covers services and supplies (including drugs and biologicals that cannot be self-administered) incident to a nurse practitioner's services that meet the requirements in paragraph (c) of this section. These services and supplies are covered only if they—

(1)   Would be covered if furnished by a physician or as incident to the professional services of a physician;

(2)   Are of the type that are commonly furnished in a physician's office and are either furnished without charge or are included in the bill for the nurse practitioner's services;

(3)   Although incidental, are an integral part of the professional service performed by the nurse practitioner; and

(4)   Are performed under the direct supervision of the nurse practitioner (that is, the nurse practitioner must be physically present and immediately available).

(e)   *Professional services.* Nurse practitioners can be paid for professional services only when the services have been personally performed by them and no facility or other provider charges, or is paid, any amount for the furnishing of the professional services.

(1)   Supervision of other nonphysician staff by a nurse practitioner does not constitute personal performance of a professional service by a nurse practitioner.

(2)   The services are provided on an assignment-related basis, and a nurse practitioner may not charge a beneficiary for a service not payable under this provision. If a beneficiary has made payment for a service, the nurse practitioner must make the appropriate refund to the beneficiary.

63 FR 58907, Nov. 2, 1998; as corrected at 64 FR 25457, May 12, 1999; as amended at 64 FR 59439, Nov. 2, 1999

Appendix A.2

42 CFR §410.76
Clinical nurse specialists' services.

(a) *Definition.* As used in this section, the term "physician" means a doctor of medicine or osteopathy, as set forth in section [1861(r)(1)] 1861(r)(1) of the Act.

(b) *Qualifications.* For Medicare Part B coverage of his or her services, a clinical nurse specialist must—

(1) Be a registered nurse who is currently licensed to practice in the State where he or she practices and be authorized to perform the services of a clinical nurse specialist in accordance with State law;

(2) Have a master's degree in a defined clinical area of nursing from an accredited educational institution; and

(3) Be certified as a clinical nurse specialist by the American Nurses Credentialing Center.

(c) *Services.* Medicare Part B covers clinical nurse specialists' services in all settings in both rural and urban areas only if the services would be covered if furnished by a physician and the clinical nurse specialist—

(1) Is legally authorized to perform them in the State in which they are performed;

(2) Is not performing services that are otherwise excluded from coverage by one of the statutory exclusions; and

(3) Performs them while working in collaboration with a physician.

(i) Collaboration is a process in which a clinical nurse specialist works with one or more physicians to deliver health care services within the scope of the practitioner's expertise, with medical direction and appropriate supervision as provided for in jointly developed guidelines or other mechanisms as provided by the law of the State in which the services are performed.

(ii) In the absence of State law governing collaboration, collaboration is a process in which a clinical nurse specialist has a relationship with one or more physicians to deliver health care services. Such collaboration is to be evidenced by clinical nurse specialists documenting the clinical nurse specialists' scope of practice and indicating the relationships that they have with physicians to deal with issues outside their scope of practice. Clinical nurse specialists must document this collaborative process with physicians.

(iii) The collaborating physician does not need to be present with the clinical nurse specialist when the services are furnished, or to make an independent evaluation of each patient who is seen by the clinical nurse specialist.

(d) *Services and supplies furnished incident to clinical nurse specialists' services.* Medicare Part B covers services and supplies (including drugs and biologicals that cannot be self-administered) incident to a clinical nurse specialist's services that meet the requirements in paragraph (c) of this section. These services and supplies are covered only if they—

(1) Would be covered if furnished by a physician or as incident to the professional services of a physician;

(2) Are of the type that are commonly furnished in a physician's office and are either furnished without charge or are included in the bill for the clinical nurse specialist's services;

(3) Although incidental, are an integral part of the professional service performed by the clinical nurse specialist; and

(4) Are performed under the direct supervision of the clinical nurse specialist (that is, the clinical nurse specialist must be physically present and immediately available).

(e) *Professional services.* Clinical nurse specialists can be paid for professional services only when the services have been personally performed by them and no facility or other provider charges, or is paid, any amount for the furnishing of the professional services.

(1) Supervision of other nonphysician staff by clinical nurse specialists does not constitute personal performance of a professional service by clinical nurse specialists.

(2) The services are provided on an assignment-related basis, and a clinical nurse specialist may not charge a beneficiary for a service not payable under this provision. If a beneficiary has made payment for a service, the clinical nurse specialist must make the appropriate refund to the beneficiary.

63 FR 58907, Nov. 2, 1998

Appendix A.3

42 CFR §410.77
Certified nurse-midwives' services: Qualifications and conditions.

(a) *Qualifications.* For Medicare coverage of his or her services, a certified nurse-midwife must:

(1)   Be a registered nurse who is legally authorized to practice as a nurse-midwife in the State where services are performed;

(2)   Have successfully completed a program of study and clinical experience for nurse-midwives that is accredited by an accrediting body approved by the U.S. Department of Education; and

(3)   Be certified as a nurse-midwife by the American College of Nurse-Midwives or the American College of Nurse-Midwives Certification Council.

(b)   *Services.* A certified nurse-midwife's services are services furnished by a certified nurse-midwife and services and supplies furnished as an incident to the certified nurse-midwife's services that—

(1)   Are within the scope of practice authorized by the law of the State in which they are furnished and would otherwise be covered if furnished by a physician or as an incident to a physician's service; and

(2)   Unless required by State law, are provided without regard to whether the certified nurse-midwife is under the supervision of, or associated with, a physician or other health care provider.

(c)   *Incident to services:* Basic rule. Medicare covers services and supplies furnished incident to the services of a certified nurse-midwife, including drugs and biologicals that cannot be self-administered, if the services and supplies meet the following conditions:

(1)   They would be covered if furnished by a physician or as incident to the professional services of a physician.

(2)   They are of the type that are commonly furnished in a physician's office and are either furnished without charge or are included in the bill for the certified nurse-midwife's services.

(3)   Although incidental, they are an integral part of the professional service performed by the certified nurse-midwife.

(4)   They are furnished under the direct supervision of a certified nurse-midwife (that is, the midwife is physically present and immediately available).

(d)   *Professional services.* A nurse-midwife can be paid for professional services only when the services have been performed personally by the nurse-midwife.

(1)   Supervision of other nonphysician staff by a nurse-midwife does not constitute personal performance of a professional service by the nurse-midwife.

(2)   The service is provided on an assignment-related basis, and a nurse-midwife may not charge a beneficiary for a service not payable under this provision. If the beneficiary has made payment for a service, the nurse-midwife must make the appropriate refund to the beneficiary.

(3)   A nurse-midwife may provide services that he or she is legally authorized to perform under State law as a nurse-midwife, if the services would otherwise be covered by the Medicare program when furnished by a physician or incident to a physicians' professional services.

63 FR 58907, Nov. 2, 1998

Appendix A.4

42 CFR §410.69
Services of a certified registered nurse anesthetist or an anesthesiologist's assistant: Basic rule and definitions.

(a) *Basic rule.* Medicare Part B pays for anesthesia services and related care furnished by a certified registered nurse anesthetist or an anesthesiologist's assistant who is legally authorized to perform the services by the State in which the services are furnished.

(b) *Definitions.* For purposes of this part—Anesthesiologist's assistant means a person who—

(1) Works under the direction of an anesthesiologist;

(2) Is in compliance with all applicable requirements of State law, including any licensure requirements the State imposes on nonphysician anesthetists; and

(3) Is a graduate of a medical school-based anesthesiologist's assistant educational program that—

(A) Is accredited by the Committee on Allied Health Education and Accreditation; and

(B) Includes approximately two years of specialized basic science and clinical education in anesthesia at a level that builds on a premedical undergraduate science background.

Anesthetist includes both an anesthesiologist's assistant and a certified registered nurse anesthetist. **Certified registered nurse anesthetist means a registered nurse who:**

(1) Is licensed as a registered professional nurse by the State in which the nurse practices;

(2) Meets any licensure requirements the State imposes with respect to non-physician anesthetists;

(3) Has graduated from a nurse anesthesia educational program that meets the standards of the Council on Accreditation of Nurse Anesthesia Programs, or such other accreditation organization as may be designated by the Secretary; and

(4) Meets the following criteria:

(i) Has passed a certification examination of the Council on Certification of Nurse Anesthetists, the Council on Recertification of Nurse Anesthetists, or any other certification organization that may be designated by the Secretary; or

(ii) Is a graduate of a program described in paragraph (3) of this definition and within 24 months after that graduation meets the requirements of paragraph (4)(i) of this definition.

57 FR 33896, July 31, 1992

Appendix A.5

42 CFR §414.56

Payment for nurse practitioners' and clinical nurse specialists' services.

(a) *Rural areas.* For services furnished beginning January 1, 1992 and ending December 31, 1997, allowed amounts for the services of a nurse practitioner or a clinical nurse specialist in a rural area (as described in section [1861(s)(2)(K)(iii)] 1861(s)(2)(K)(iii) of the Act) may not exceed the following limits:

(1) For services furnished in a hospital (including assistant-at-surgery services), 75 percent of the physician fee schedule amount for the service.

(2) For all other services, 85 percent of the physician fee schedule amount for the service.

(b) *Non-rural areas.* For services furnished beginning January 1, 1992 and ending December 31, 1997, allowed amounts for the services of a nurse practitioner or a clinical nurse specialist in a nursing facility may not exceed 85 percent of the physician fee schedule amount for the service.

(c) Beginning January 1, 1998. For services (other than assistant-at-surgery services) furnished beginning January 1, 1998, allowed amounts for the services of a nurse practitioner or clinical nurse specialist may not exceed 85 percent of the physician fee schedule amount for the service. For assistant-at-surgery services, allowed amounts for the services of a nurse practitioner or clinical nurse specialist may not exceed 85 percent of the physician fee schedule amount that would be allowed under the physician fee schedule if the assistant-at-surgery service were furnished by a physician.

56 FR 59624, Nov. 25, 1991, as amended at 57 FR 42493, Sept. 15, 1992; 63 FR 58911, Nov. 2, 1998

Appendix A.6

42 CFR §414.54
Payment for certified nurse-midwives' services.

For services furnished after December 31, 1991, allowed amounts under the fee schedule established under section [1833(a)(1)(K)] 1833(a)(1)(K) of the Act for the payment of certified nurse-midwife services may not exceed 65 percent of the physician fee schedule amount for the service.

Appendix A.7

42 CFR §414.60

Payment for the services of CRNAs.

(a) *Basis for payment.* The allowance for the anesthesia service furnished by a CRNA, medically directed or not medically directed, is based on allowable base and time units as defined in §414.46(a).

Beginning with CY 1994—

(1) The allowance for an anesthesia service furnished by a medically directed CRNA is based on a fixed percentage of the allowance recognized for the anesthesia service personally performed by the physician alone, as specified in §414.46(d)(3); and

(2) The CF for an anesthesia service furnished by a CRNA not directed by a physician may not exceed the CF for a service personally performed by a physician.

(b) *To whom payment may be made.* Payment for an anesthesia service furnished by a CRNA may be made to the CRNA or to any individual or entity (such as a hospital, critical access hospital, physician, group practice, or ambulatory surgical center) with which the CRNA has an employment or contract relationship that provides for payment to be made to the individual or entity.

(c) *Condition for payment.* Payment for the services of a CRNA may be made only on an assignment related basis, and any assignment accepted by a CRNA is binding on any other person presenting a claim or request for payment for the service.

60 FR 63178, Dec. 8, 1995, as amended at 62 FR 46037, Aug. 29, 1997; 64 FR 59441, Nov. 2, 1999

Appendix A.7

42 CFR §414.46
Additional rules for payment of anesthesia services.

(a) *Definitions.* For purposes of this section, the following definitions apply:

(1) Base unit means the value for each anesthesia code that reflects all activities other than anesthesia time. These activities include usual preoperative and postoperative visits, the administration of fluids and blood incident to anesthesia care, and monitoring services.

(2) Anesthesia practitioner, for the purpose of anesthesia time, means a physician who performs the anesthesia service alone, a CRNA who is not medically directed who performs the anesthesia service alone, or a medically directed CRNA.

(3) Anesthesia time means the time during which an anesthesia practitioner is present with the patient. It starts when the anesthesia practitioner begins to prepare the patient for anesthesia services and ends when the anesthesia practitioner is no longer furnishing anesthesia services to the beneficiary, that is, when the beneficiary may be placed safely under postoperative care. Anesthesia time is a continuous time period from the start of anesthesia to the end of an anesthesia service. In counting anesthesia time, the anesthesia practitioner can add blocks of anesthesia time around an interruption in anesthesia time as long as the anesthesia practitioner is furnishing continuous anesthesia care within the time periods around the interruption.

(b) *Determination of payment amount—Basic rule.* For anesthesia services performed, medically directed, or medically supervised by a physician, HCFA pays the lesser of the actual charge or the anesthesia fee schedule amount.

(1) The carrier bases the fee schedule amount for an anesthesia service on the product of the sum of allowable base and time units and an anesthesia-specific CF. The carrier calculates the time units from the anesthesia time reported by the anesthesia practitioner for the anesthesia procedure. The physician who fulfills the conditions for medical direction in §415.110 (Conditions for payment: Anesthesiology services) reports the same anesthesia time as the medically-directed CRNA.

(2) HCFA furnishes the carrier with the base units for each anesthesia procedure code. The base units are derived from the 1988 American Society of Anesthesiologists' Relative Value Guide except that the number of base units recognized for anesthesia services furnished during cataract or iridectomy surgery is four units.

(3) Modifier units are not allowed. Modifier units include additional units charged by a physician or a CRNA for patient health status, risk, age, or unusual circumstances.

(c) Physician personally performs the anesthesia procedure.

(1) HCFA considers an anesthesia service to be personally performed under any of the following circumstances:

(i) The physician performs the entire anesthesia service alone.

(ii) The physician establishes an attending physician relationship in one or two concurrent cases involving an intern or resident and the service was furnished before January 1, 1994.

(iii) The physician establishes an attending physician relationship in one case involving an intern or resident and the service was furnished on or after January 1, 1994 but prior to January 1, 1996. For services on or after January 1, 1996, the physician must be the teaching physician as defined in §§ 415.170 through 415.184 of this chapter.

(iv) The physician and the CRNA or AA are involved in a single case and the services of each are found to be medically necessary.

(v) The physician is continuously involved in a single case involving a student nurse anesthetist.

(vi) The physician is continuously involved in a single case involving a CRNA or AA and the service was furnished prior to January 1, 1998.

(2) HCFA determines the fee schedule amount for an anesthesia service personally performed by a physician on the basis of an anesthesia-specific fee schedule CF and unreduced base units and anesthesia time units. One anesthesia time unit is equivalent to 15 minutes of anesthesia time, and fractions of a 15-minute period are recognized as fractions of an anesthesia time unit.

(d) Anesthesia services medically directed by a physician.

(1) HCFA considers an anesthesia service to be medically directed by a physician if:

(i) The physician performs the activities described in §415.110 of this chapter.

(ii) The physician directs qualified individuals involved in two, three, or four concurrent cases.

(iii) Medical direction can occur for a single case furnished on or after January 1, 1998 if the physician performs the activities described in §415.110 of this chapter and medically directs a single CRNA or AA.

(2) The rules for medical direction differ for certain time periods depending on the nature of the qualified individual who is directed by the physician. If more than two procedures are directed on or after January 1, 1994, the qualified individuals could be AAs, CRNAs, interns, or residents. The medical direction rules apply to student nurse anesthetists only if the physician directs two concurrent cases, each of which involves a student nurse anesthetist or the physician directs one case involving a student nurse anesthetist and the other involving a CRNA, AA, intern, or resident.

(3) Payment for medical direction is based on a specific percentage of the payment allowance recognized for the anesthesia service personally performed by a physician alone. The following percentages apply for the years specified:

(i) CY 1994—60 percent of the payment allowance for personally performed procedures.

(ii) CY 1995—57.5 percent of the payment allowance for personally performed services.

(iii) CY 1996—55 percent of the payment allowance for personally performed services.

(iv) CY 1997—52.5 percent of the payment allowance for personally performed services.

(v) CY 1998 and thereafter—50 percent of the payment allowance for personally performed services.

(e) Physician medically supervises anesthesia services. If the physician medically supervises more than four concurrent anesthesia services, HCFA bases the fee schedule amount on an anesthesia-specific CF and three base units. This represents payment for the physician's involvement in the pre-surgical anesthesia services.

(f) Payment for medical or surgical services furnished by a physician while furnishing anesthesia services.

    (1) HCFA allows separate payment under the fee schedule for certain reasonable and medically necessary medical or surgical services furnished by a physician while furnishing anesthesia services to the patient. HCFA makes payment for these services in accordance with the general physician fee schedule rules in §414.20. These services are described in program operating instructions.

    (2) HCFA makes no separate payment for other medical or surgical services, such as the pre-anesthetic examination of the patient, pre- or post-operative visits, or usual monitoring functions, that are ordinarily included in the anesthesia service.

(g) Physician involved in multiple anesthesia services. If the physician is involved in multiple anesthesia services for the same patient during the same operative session, the carrier makes payment according to the base unit associated with the anesthesia service having the highest base unit value and anesthesia time that encompasses the multiple services.

56 FR 59624, Nov. 25, 1991, as amended at 57 FR 42492, Sept. 15, 1992; 58 FR 63687, Dec. 2, 1993; 60 FR 63177, Dec. 8, 1995; 64 FR 59441, Nov. 2, 1999.

Appendix A.9

42 CFR §414.52

Payment for physician assistants' services.

Allowed amounts for the services of a physician assistant furnished beginning January 1, 1992 and ending December 31, 1997, may not exceed the limits specified in paragraphs (a) through (c) of this section. Allowed amounts for the services of a physician assistant furnished beginning January 1, 1998, may not exceed the limits specified in paragraph (d) of this section.

(a) For assistant-at-surgery services, 65 percent of the amount that would be allowed under the physician fee schedule if the assistant-at-surgery service was furnished by a physician.

(b) For services (other than assistant-at-surgery services) furnished in a hospital, 75 percent of the physician fee schedule amount for the service.

(c) For all other services, 85 percent of the physician fee schedule amount for the service.

(d) For services (other than assistant-at-surgery services) furnished beginning January 1, 1998, 85 percent of the physician fee schedule amount for the service. For assistant-at-surgery services, 85 percent of the physician fee schedule amount that would be allowed under the physician fee schedule if the assistant-at-surgery service were furnished by a physician.

63 FR 58911, Nov. 2, 1998

Appendix A.10

42 CFR §410.32
Diagnostic X-ray tests, diagnostic laboratory tests, and other diagnostic tests: Conditions.

(a) *Ordering diagnostic tests.* All diagnostic x-ray tests, diagnostic laboratory tests, and other diagnostic tests must be ordered by the physician who is treating the beneficiary, that is, the physician who furnishes a consultation or treats a beneficiary for a specific medical problem and who uses the results in the management of the beneficiary's specific medical, problem. Tests not ordered by the physician who is treating the beneficiary are not reasonable and necessary (see [sect] 411.15(k)(1) of this chapter).

(1) Chiropractic exception. A physician may order an x-ray to be used by a chiropractor to demonstrate the subluxation of the spine that is the basis for a beneficiary to receive manual manipulation treatments even though the physician does not treat the beneficiary.

(2) Mammography exception. A physician who meets the qualification requirements for an interpreting physician under section 354 of the Public Health Service Act as provided in [sect] 410.34(a)(7) may order a diagnostic mammogram based on the findings of a screening mammogram even though the physician does not treat the beneficiary.

(3) Application to nonphysician practitioners. Nonphysician practitioners (that is, clinical nurse specialists, clinical psychologists, clinical social workers, nurse-midwives, nurse practitioners, and physician assistants) who furnish services that would be physician services if furnished by a physician, and who are operating within the scope of their authority under State law and within the scope of their Medicare statutory benefit, may be treated the same as physicians treating beneficiaries for the purpose of this paragraph.

(b) *Diagnostic x-ray and other diagnostic tests.*

(1) Basic rule. Except as indicated in paragraph (b)(2) of this section, all diagnostic x-ray and other diagnostic tests covered under section 1861(s)(3) of the Act and payable under the physician fee schedule must be furnished under the appropriate level of supervision by a physician as defined in section1861(r) of the Act. Services furnished without the required level of supervision are not reasonable and necessary (see [sect] 411.15(k)(1) of this chapter).

(2) Exceptions. The following diagnostic tests payable under the physician fee schedule are excluded from the basic rule set forth in paragraph (b)(1) of this section:

(i) Diagnostic mammography procedures, which are regulated by the Food and Drug Administration.

(ii) Diagnostic tests personally furnished by a qualified audiologist as defined in section 1861(11)(3) of the Act.

(iii) Diagnostic psychological testing services personally furnished by a clinical psychologist or a qualified independent psychologist as defined in program instructions.

(iv) Diagnostic tests (as established through program instructions) personally performed by a physical therapist who is certified by the American Board of Physical Therapy Specialties as a qualified electrophysiologic clinical specialist and permitted to provide the service under State law.

(v) Diagnostic tests performed by a nurse practitioner or clinical nurse specialist authorized to perform the tests under applicable State laws.

(vi) Pathology and laboratory procedures listed in the 80000 series of the Current Procedural Terminology published by the American Medical Association.

(3) Levels of supervision. Except where otherwise indicated, all diagnostic x-ray and other diagnostic tests subject to this provision and payable under the physician fee schedule must be furnished under at least a general level of physician supervision as defined in paragraph (b)(3)(i) of this section. In addition, some of these tests also require either direct or personal supervision as defined in paragraphs (b)(3)(ii) or (b)(3)(iii) of this section, respectively. (However, diagnostic tests performed by a physician assistant (PA) that the PA is legally authorized to perform under State law require only a general level of physician supervision.) When direct or personal supervision is required, physician supervision at the specified level is required throughout the performance of the test.

(i) General supervision means the procedure is furnished under the physician's overall direction and control, but the physician's presence is not required during the performance of the procedure. Under general supervision, the training of the nonphysician personnel who actually perform the diagnostic procedure and the maintenance of the necessary equipment and supplies are the continuing responsibility of the physician.

(ii) Direct supervision in the office setting means the physician must be present in the office suite and immediately available to furnish assistance and direction throughout the performance of the procedure. It does not mean that the physician must be present in the room when the procedure is performed.

(iii) Personal supervision means a physician must be in attendance in the room during the performance of the procedure.

(c) *Portable x-ray services.* Portable x-ray services furnished in a place of residence used as the patient's home are covered if the following conditions are met:

(1) These services are furnished under the general supervision of a physician, as defined in paragraph (b)(3)(i) of this section.

(2) The supplier of these services meets the requirements set forth in part 486, subpart C of this chapter, concerning conditions for coverage for portable x-ray services.

(3) The procedures are limited to

(i) Skeletal films involving the extremities, pelvis, vertebral column, or skull;

(ii) Chest or abdominal films that do not involve the use of contrast media; and

(iii) Diagnostic mammograms if the approved portable x-ray supplier, as defined in subpart C of part 486 of this chapter, meets the certification requirements of section 354 of the Public Health Service Act, as implemented by 21 CFR part 900, subpart B.

(d) *Diagnostic laboratory tests.* Medicare Part B pays for covered diagnostic laboratory tests that are furnished by any of the following;

(1) A participating hospital or participating RPCH.

(2) A nonparticipating hospital that meets the requirements for emergency outpatient services specified in subpart G of part 424 of this chapter and the laboratory requirements specified in part 493 of this chapter.

(3) The office of the patient's attending or consulting physician if that physician is a doctor of medicine, osteopathy, podiatric medicine, dental surgery, or dental medicine.

(4) An RHC.

(5) A laboratory, if it meets the applicable requirements for laboratories of part 493 of this chapter, including the laboratory of a nonparticipating hospital that does not meet the requirements for emergency outpatient services in subpart G of [42 CFR 424] part 424 of this chapter.

(6) An FQHC.

(7) An SNF to its resident under § 411.15(p) of this chapter, either directly (in accordance with § 483.75(k)(1)(i) of this chapter) or under an arrangement (as defined in § 409.3 of this chapter) with another entity described in this paragraph.

64 FR 59439, Nov. 2, 1999

Appendix A.11

42 CFR §410.33

Independent diagnostic testing facility.

(a) *General rule.*

(1) Effective for diagnostic procedures performed on or after March 15, 1999, carriers will pay for diagnostic procedures under the physician fee schedule only when performed by a physician, a group practice of physicians, an approved supplier of portable x-ray services, a nurse practitioner, or a clinical nurse specialist when he or she performs a test he or she is authorized by the State to perform, or an independent diagnostic testing facility (IDTF). An IDTF may be a fixed location, a mobile entity, or an individual nonphysician practitioner. It is independent of a physician's office or hospital; however, these rules apply when an IDTF furnishes diagnostic procedures in a physician's office.

(2) Exceptions. The following diagnostic tests that are payable under the physician fee schedule and furnished by a nonhospital testing entity are not required to be furnished in accordance with the criteria set forth in paragraphs (b) through (e) of this section:

(i) Diagnostic mammography procedures, which are regulated by the Food and Drug Administration.

(ii) Diagnostic tests personally furnished by a qualified audiologist as defined in section 1861(ll)(3) of the Act.

(iii) Diagnostic psychological testing services personally furnished by a clinical psychologist or a qualified independent psychologist as defined in program instructions.

(iv) Diagnostic tests (as established through program instructions) personally performed by a physical therapist who is certified by the American Board of Physical Therapy Specialties as a qualified electrophysiologic clinical specialist and permitted to provide the service under State law.

(b) *Supervising physician.*

(1) An IDTF must have one or more supervising physicians who are responsible for the direct and ongoing oversight of the quality of the testing performed, the proper operation and calibration of the equipment used to perform tests, and the qualification of nonphysician personnel who use the equipment. This level of supervision is that required for general supervision set forth in [sect] 410.32(b)(3)(i).

(2) The supervising physician must evidence proficiency in the performance and interpretation of each type of diagnostic procedure performed by the IDTF. The proficiency may be documented by certification in specific medical specialties or subspecialties or by criteria established by the carrier for the service area in which the IDTF is located. In the case of a procedure requiring the direct or personal supervision of a physician as set forth in [sect] 410.32(b)(3)(ii) or (b)(3)(iii), the IDTF's supervising physician must personally furnish this level of supervision whether the procedure is performed in the IDTF or, in the case of mobile services, at the remote location. The IDTF must maintain documentation of sufficient physician resources during all hours of operations to assure that the required physician supervision is

furnished. In the case of procedures requiring direct supervision, the supervising physician may oversee concurrent procedures.

(c) *Nonphysician personnel.* Any nonphysician personnel used by the IDTF to perform tests must demonstrate the basic qualifications to perform the tests in question and have training and proficiency as evidenced by licensure or certification by the appropriate state health or education department. In the absence of a State licensing board, the technician must be certified by an appropriate national credentialing body. The IDTF must maintain documentation available for review that these requirements are met.

(d) *Ordering of tests.* All procedures performed by the IDTF must be specifically ordered in writing by the physician who is treating the beneficiary, that is, the physician who is furnishing a consultation or treating a beneficiary for a specific medical problem and who uses the results in the management of the beneficiary's specific medical problem.

(Nonphysician practitioners may order tests as set forth in [sect] 410.32(a)(3).) The order must specify the diagnosis or other basis for the testing. The supervising physician for the IDTF may not order tests to be performed by the IDTF, unless the IDTF's supervising physician is in fact the beneficiary's treating physician. That is, the physician in question had a relationship with the beneficiary prior to the performance of the testing and is treating the beneficiary for a specific, medical problem. The IDTF may not add any procedures based on internal protocols without a written order from the treating physician.

(e) *Multi-State entities.* An IDTF that operates across State boundaries must maintain documentation that its supervising physicians and technicians are licensed and certified in each of the States in which it is furnishing services.

(f) *Applicability of State law.* An IDTF must comply with the applicable laws of any State in which it operates.

62 FR 59099, Oct. 31, 1997, as amended at 64 FR 59439, Nov. 2, 1999

Appendix A.12

42 CFR §410.78
Consultations via telecommunications systems.

(a) *General rule.* Medicare Part B pays for professional consultations furnished by means of interactive telecommunications systems if the following conditions are met:

(1) The consulting practitioner is any of the following:

(i) A physician as described in §410.20.

(ii) A physician assistant as defined in §410.74.

(iii) A nurse practitioner as defined in §410.75

(iv) A clinical nurse specialist as described in §410.76.

(v) A nurse-midwife as defined in §410.77.

(2) The referring practitioner is any of the following:

(i) A physician as described in §410.20.

(ii) A physician assistant as defined in §410.74.

(iii) A nurse practitioner as defined in §410.75.

(iv) A clinical nurse specialist as described in §410.76.

(v) A nurse-midwife as defined in §410.77.

(vi) A clinical psychologist as described at §410.71.

(vii) A clinical social worker as defined in §410.73.

(3) The services are furnished to a beneficiary residing in a rural area as defined in section 1886(d)(2)(D) of the Act, and the area is designated as a health professional shortage area (HPSA) under section 332(a)(1)(A) of the Public Health Service Act (42 U.S.C. 254e(a)(1)(A). For purposes of this requirement, the beneficiary is deemed to be residing in such an area if the teleconsultation presentation takes place in such an area.

(4) The medical examination of the beneficiary is under the control of the consulting practitioner.

(5) As a condition of payment, the teleconsultation involves the participation of the referring practitioner, or a practitioner described in section 1842(b)(18)(C) of the Act (other than a certified registered nurse anesthetist or anesthesiologist assistant) who is an employee of the referring practitioner, as appropriate to the medical needs of the patient and as needed to provide information to and at the direction of the consultant.

(6) The consultation results in a written report that is furnished to the referring practitioner.

(b) *Definition.* For purposes of this section, interactive telecommunications systems means multimedia communications equipment that includes, at a minimum, audio and video equipment permitting real-time consultation among the patient, consultant, and referring practitioner, or a practitioner described in section [1842(b)(18)(C)] 1842(b)(18)(C) of the Act (other than a certified registered nurse anesthetist or anesthesiologist assistant) who is an employee of the referring practitioner, as appropriate to the medical needs of the patient and as needed to provide information to and at the direction of the consulting practitioner. Telephones, facsimile machines, and electronic mail systems do not meet the definition of interactive telecommunications systems.

63 FR 58907, Nov. 2, 1998

Appendix B

Medicare Forms

> The copies of the forms in this appendix are provided for reference only.
> They are not intended for reproduction in any form.

1. Medicare Health Care Provider/Supplier Application (HCFA 855)
2. Medicare Change of Enrollment Information Form (HCFA 855C)
3. Medicare Health Insurance Claim Form (HCFA 1500)
4. HCFA 1500 Claim Form Instructions
5. Individual Reassignment of Benefits Application (HCFA 855R)

OMB Approval No. 0938-0685

MEDICARE
AND OTHER FEDERAL HEALTH CARE PROGRAM
GENERAL ENROLLMENT

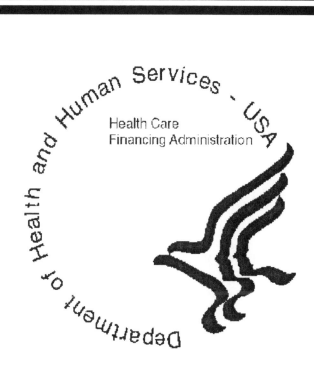

Health Care
Financing Administration

Department of Health and Human Services - USA

Health Care
Provider/Supplier Application

HCFA 855 (1/98)

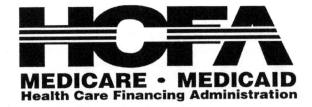

MEDICARE AND OTHER FEDERAL HEALTH CARE PROGRAMS PROVIDER/SUPPLIER ENROLLMENT APPLICATION INSTRUCTIONS
General Application - HCFA 855

Upon completion, return this application and all necessary documentation to:

General

This application must be completed by all providers and suppliers of medical and other health services for enrollment in the Medicare or any other federal health care program.

Some applicants may also need to be surveyed and/or certified by the appropriate State Agency or Regional Medicare Office when required to meet Medicare conditions of enrollment. In this case, those applicants must initially contact the State Agency or Regional Medicare Office prior to completion and submission of this application.

If you need assistance or have any questions concerning the completion of this application, contact your local Medicare or other federal health care contractor.

A separate application must be submitted for each classification of provider/supplier type (e.g., physician in private practice, physician in group practice) even if the different types of services are furnished within the same organization or entity (e.g., hospitals and all affiliated units).

Each entity of an organization must submit a separate application (e.g., hospital based skilled nursing facility, hospices, outpatient clinics, etc.). Each entity of a chain organization must submit a separate application.

Providers and/or suppliers enrolling in the Medicare or any other federal health care program as a group member, partner, or individual contractor who reassigns their Medicare or other federal health care program benefits to the enrolling applicant must also complete HCFA Form 855R (Individual Reassignment of Benefits Application).

Suppliers of Durable Medical Equipment, Prosthetics, Orthotics, and Supplies must enroll in the Medicare or any other federal health care program using HCFA Form 855S (DMEPOS Supplier Enrollment Application) instead of this application.

Upon completion and approval of this application, the applicant will be issued a provider/supplier billing number. This number will be automatically deactivated if it is inactive for 12 consecutive months. A new HCFA Form 855 must be completed and approved to re-activate the billing number.

For your convenience, the application form of this package has been perforated for easy removal of individual pages. It is not necessary to return the instructions or unused attachments when returning this completed application.

Note: Any changes in the information reported in this application must be reported to the Medicare or other federal health care contractor within <u>30 calendar days</u> of said change.

Definitions

Authorized Representative: The appointed official (e.g., officer, chief executive officer, general partner, etc.) who has the authority to enroll the entity in Medicare or other federal health care programs as well as to make changes and/or updates to the applicant's status, and to commit the corporation to Medicare or other federal health care program laws and regulations.

The Authorized Representative may be contacted to answer questions regarding the information furnished in this application.

Chain Organization: Multiple providers and/or suppliers (chains) are owned, leased or through any other devices, controlled by a single business entity. The chain organization must consist of two or more health care facilities. The controlling business entity is called the chain "Home Office." Each entity in the chain may have a different owner (generally chains are not owned by the "Home Office").

Typically, the chain "Home Office:"

> -maintains uniform procedures in each facility for handling admissions, utilization review, preparation and processing admission notices and bills;

> -maintains and controls centrally, individual provider/supplier cost reports and fiscal records and a major part of the Medicare audit for each component can be performed centrally.

Examples of provider types that would typically be chain organizations are: Certified Outpatient Rehabilitation Facilities (CORFs); Skilled Nursing Facilities (SNFs); and Home Health Agencies (HHAs).

Clinical Laboratory Improvement Amendments (CLIA) Number : This number is assigned to laboratories who are certified by the Health Care Financing Administration (HCFA) under the Clinical Laboratory Improvement Amendments.

> **Note:** Any laboratory soliciting or accepting specimens for laboratory testing is required to hold a valid certificate issued by the Secretary of the United States Department of Health and Human Services or hold a license from a CLIA exempt State.

Consolidated Cost Report: A cost report compiled for multiple facilities joined together and filed under the parent facility's Medicare Identification Number.

Contractor: Any individual, entity, facility, organization, business, group practice, etc., receiving an Internal Revenue Service (IRS) Form 1099 for services provided to this applicant (e.g., independent contractor, subcontractor).

Distinct Part Unit [of a facility]: A separate psychiatric, rehabilitation, or skilled nursing unit that is attached to a hospital paid under the Prospective Payment System (PPS) but which is paid on a cost reimbursement or other non-PPS basis. It must be a clearly identifiable unit, such as an entire ward, wing, floor, or building, including all the beds and related services in the unit, that meets all the requirements for a type of facility other than the one in which it is located, **and** houses all the beneficiaries and recipients for whom payment is made under Medicare for services in the other type of facility.

Food and Drug Administration Number (FDA): This is the certification number assigned by the FDA for equipment used in mammography screening and diagnostic services.

Group Member: A physician or non-physician practitioner who renders services in a group practice and who reassigns benefits to the group.

Independent Diagnostic Testing Facility (IDTF) (formerly Independent Physiological Laboratories (IPL's)): An entity independent of a hospital or physician's office in which diagnostic tests are performed by licensed, certified non-physician personnel under appropriate physician supervision (e.g., free standing cardiac catherization facility, imaging center, etc.).

Legal Business Name: The legal name of the individual or entity applying for enrollment. This name should be the same name the applicant uses in reporting to the Internal Revenue Service.

Medicaid Number: This number uniquely identifies the applicant as a Medicaid provider and/or supplier in a given State.

Medicare Identification Number: This number uniquely identifies the applicant as a Medicare provider and/or supplier and is the number used on claim forms. The Medicare Identification Number is also known as Medicare Provider Number and Provider Identification Number (PIN). Examples of Medicare Identification Numbers are the UPINs, OSCAR numbers, and NSC numbers.

> **Note:** If the applicant is enrolling in the Medicare or other federal health care programs for the first time, the applicant will receive a Medicare or other federal health care program identification number upon enrollment.

National Provider Identifier (NPI): This number is assigned using the National Provider System to identify health care providers and/or suppliers. In the future, it will replace the Medicare Identification Number.

National Supplier Clearinghouse Number (NSC): This number uniquely identifies the applicant as a supplier of durable medical equipment, prosthetics, orthotics and supplies (DMEPOS). It is the number used by DMEPOS suppliers on claim forms.

On-Line Survey Certification and Reporting System (OSCAR): National database used for maintaining and retrieving survey and certification data for certified providers and/or suppliers that are approved to participate in the Medicare, Medicaid and CLIA programs. OSCAR numbers are assigned by the Regional Medicare office.

Other Affiliated Units: Entities that are either a Provider Based Facility, a Distinct Part Unit, or file a consolidated cost report.

Provider Based Facility: Entities operating under the control of a parent organization (e.g., hospital based End Stage Renal Disease Unit, Skilled Nursing Facility, etc.).

Reassignee: An individual or organization that allows another organization to bill Medicare or other federal health care programs on their behalf for services rendered.

Unique Physician Identification Number (UPIN): This number is assigned to physicians, non-physician practitioners and groups to identify the referring or ordering physician on Medicare claims.

APPLICATION COMPLETION INSTRUCTIONS

Furnish all requested information in its entirety. If a field is not applicable, write N/A in the field. If entire section is not applicable, check the box at the beginning of the section indicating the entire section is not applicable. Any section of the application that does <u>not</u> have a check box at the beginning of the section indicating the entire section is not applicable <u>must</u> be completed by applicant.

Check Type of Business: (For administrative purposes only)

Check appropriate box indicating how applicant's business is structured. The answer to this item will not affect the amount of reimbursement or enrollment status.

> **Note:** If applicant's business structure is a **partnership,** applicant must provide a copy of its partnership agreement signed by all parties and identifying the general partner (if any) and attest that the partnership meets all State requirements. **Partnerships** see group instruction.

Check "Applicant Enrolling As" Type: (For administrative purposes only)   The answer to this item will not affect the amount of reimbursement or enrollment status.

See the instructions below that identify which sections the applicant is responsible for completing.

Individual: An individual person enrolling as a physician, supplier or non-physician practitioner (e.g., physician, nurse, midwife, etc.).

> **Note:** An individual who is registered as a business is considered a sole proprietor for the purpose of completing this application and should not check this box.

> **Individuals** complete sections 1a, 1d, 2, 3, 4, 5, 6, 7, 8, 9, 12, 13, 14, 15, 17, and 18.

Sole Proprietor: An individual person registered as a business and issued a tax identification number from the IRS and rendering services under the business name.

> **Sole Proprietors** complete sections 1a, 1b, 1d, 2, 3, 4, 5, 6, 7, 8, 9, 12, 13, 14, 15, 17 and 18.

Organization: A company, not-for-profit entity, governmental agency (Federal, State, or Local) or a qualified health care delivery system which renders medical care (e.g., pharmacy, equipment manufacturer, hospital, Public Health Clinic, laboratory, skilled nursing facility, Ambulance Service Supplier, Independent Diagnostic Testing Facility, etc.).

> **Organizations** complete sections 1b, 1d, 2, 5, 6, 7, 8, 9, 10, 11, 12, 13, 14, 15, 16, 17, and 18.

Ambulance Service Suppliers must also complete Attachment 1.

Independent Diagnostic Testing Facilities must also complete Attachment 2.

Home Health Agencies must also complete Attachment 3.

Group: Two or more physicians, non-physician practitioners or other health care providers/suppliers who form a practice together (as authorized by State law) and bill Medicare or other federal health care programs as a single unit. A group has individual practitioners. The individual members must be enumerated and enrolled in the Medicare or other federal health care program as individuals in order to enroll as members of the group.

Only those health care practitioners who are authorized to bill Medicare or other federal health care programs directly in their individual capacities are allowed to form a group. A group can only be enrolled if it can meet the conditions for reassignment (see instructions for the Reassignment of Benefits section).

The above definition of a group is to be used for Medicare or other federal health care programs' enrollment purposes only. It is not the group definition described in section 1877(h) of the Social Security Act.

> **Groups/Partnerships** complete sections 1b, 1c, 1d, 2, 5, 6, 7, 8, 9, 10, 11, 12, 13, 14, 15, 17 and 18.

All group member/partners must complete HCFA Form 855R.

> **Note: PARTNERSHIPS:** For purposes of this application, partnerships should check that they are "enrolling as" a group.

> **Note: RURAL HEALTH CLINICS:** Rural Health Clinics that meet the definition of a group, should also submit HCFA Form 855R (Individual Reassignment of Benefits Application) for each member of the group. This is not applicable to those Rural Health Clinics that are provider based.

Mass Immunization Biller Only: A health care provider/supplier who roster bills Medicare or other federal health care programs solely for mass immunizations.

> **Mass Immunization/Roster Billers** complete sections 1a, 1b, 1d, 2, 5, 6, 7, 8, 9, 12, 13, 14, 15, 17 and 18.

> **Note:** Applicants enrolling in the Medicare or other federal health care program as mass immunization/roster billers cannot bill the Medicare or other federal health care program for any other services. The applicant agrees to accept assignment of the influenza/pneumococcus benefit as payment in full and cannot "balance bill" the beneficiary.

> For those who are only applying to enroll in the Medicare or other federal health care program to roster bill for mass immunization, enter "Roster" under primary speciality in Section 1A if applicant is an individual, or enter "Roster" under type of facility in Section 1B if applicant is an organization.

Check appropriate federal health care program:

If applicant is enrolling in a federal health care program other than Medicare, check the appropriate box. Check only one box. For each federal health care program in which the applicant wishes to enroll, the applicant must complete a separate enrollment application and submit it to that federal health care program.

Check Application For:

Initial Enrollment: Applicant is enrolling in the Medicare or other federal health care programs for the first time, or re-activating a prior Medicare billing number.

Enrollment of Additional Location(s): Currently enrolled provider/supplier is applying to enroll a new practice location.

Recertification: Currently enrolled provider/supplier is completing application to comply with mandatory periodic re-survey and/or recertification through the State agency or Regional Medicare Office.

Change of Ownership (CHOW): This term applies to certain limited circumstances as defined in 42 CFR § 489.18 as described below.

A new or prospective new owner must complete this application to report new or prospective new ownership. In addition, the applicant must also submit an Individual Reassignment of Benefits Application (HCFA Form 855R) identifying all individuals who will reassign their benefits to the applicant.

A change of ownership is defined as:

- In the case of a <u>partnership</u>, the removal, addition, or substitution of a partner, unless the partners expressly agree otherwise, as permitted by applicable State law;

- In the case of an <u>unincorporated sole proprietorship</u>, transfer of title and property to another party;

- In the case of a <u>corporation</u>, the merger of the provider corporation into another corporation, or the consolidation of two or more corporations, resulting in the creation of a new corporation (transfer of corporate stock or the merger of another corporation into the provider corporation does not constitute a change of ownership); and

- In the case of <u>leasing</u>, the lease of all or part of a provider/supplier facility constitutes a change of ownership of the leased portion.

     Note: A currently enrolled provider/supplier who is reporting new information on the current owners (i.e., addition(s) or deletion(s) of owner(s)) which is not expected to result in a CHOW as defined above, must make the appropriate changes using the ownership information section of this application. This action is considered a change of information (see below).

Change of Information: Currently enrolled provider/supplier is completing applicable sections of the application to report a change in information other than a CHOW as defined above. Currently enrolled provider/suppliers can use HCFA Form 855C (Change of Information Form) to report changes in name, specialty, e-mail address, practice location address, billing agency address, pay to address, surety bond changes/renewals, mailing address, pricing locality, telephone number(s), fax number(s), deactivation of Medicare or other federal health care billing number(s), addition or deletion of authorized representatives, and potential termination of current ownership.

Changes not listed above must be reported using this application.

When using this application to notify the Medicare or other federal health care program that a practice location(s), owner(s), or various personnel are no longer associated with this entity, check the appropriate deletion box in the applicable section(s) and identify the practice location and/or personnel.

All changes must be reported in writing and have an original signature. For individuals, the applicant must sign and for organizations and group practices, an "Authorized Representative" must sign to confirm the requested change(s). Faxed or photocopied signatures will **not** be accepted.

Check Where Applicant Will Be Submitting Bills:

MEDICARE APPLICANTS ONLY

Fiscal Intermediary: Applicant will be enrolled to bill the fiscal intermediary only. The fiscal intermediary is generally known as the Part A Medicare Contractor. The applicant will generally be a hospital or other health care facility.

Carrier: Applicant will be enrolled to bill the carrier only. The carrier is generally known as the Part B Medicare Contractor. The applicant will generally be a physician or non-physician practitioner.

Both: Application will automatically be forwarded to bill both the fiscal intermediary and the carrier for enrollment consideration.

Regional Home Health Intermediary: Applicant will be enrolled to bill the regional home health intermediary.

If applicant checked that they will be billing a fiscal intermediary, indicate applicant's preferred choice of fiscal intermediary from the separate list included in this package.

Check other federal health care program(s) where applicant is currently enrolled:

If applicant is currently enrolled in any other federal health care program(s), check all appropriate boxes.

---

1. Applicant Identification

A. Individuals Only

Complete all items in this section if applicant plans to bill the Medicare or other federal health care program as an individual practitioner.

If an individual or sole proprietorship, complete applicant's full name (this is the name payment will be made in), date and place of birth (county and/or city). If applicant has previously practiced or operated a business under another name, including applicant's maiden name, supply that name under Other Name.

If applicable, check if applicant is a resident or intern at a hospital.

If applicant is enrolling as an individual or sole proprietor, furnish the applicant's primary speciality (e.g. general practitioner, urologist, nurse practitioner, etc.). Listing a secondary speciality is optional.

Gender and Race/Ethnicity information is optional. This data will only be used to assist HCFA in uniquely identifying the applicant.

A. Individuals Only (continued)

If applicant is employed by an entity that will receive payments for the applicant's services, applicant must complete and sign the HCFA Form 855R (Individual Reassignment of Benefits Application).

B. Organizations Only

Complete this section if applicant is a sole proprietor of the business or if applicant is a publicly or privately held business entity.

Complete all items in this section. For Legal Business Name, supply the name that the business, organization or group practice reports to the IRS (this is the name payment will be made in). For Type of Facility give the classification that designates the entity (e.g., hospital, skilled nursing facility, home health agency, ambulance company, etc.), and check whether this facility is accredited or non-accredited.

> **Note:** Clinical laboratories and independent diagnostic testing facilities should annotate this section "LABORATORY" (LAB).

All organizations must identify if they are considered a Provider Based Facility, a Distinct Part Unit, or file a consolidated cost report under another provider/supplier Medicare identification number. If an organization is a Distinct Part Unit, then the organization also falls under the broader category of Provider Based Facility.

If the organization is a:

- Provider Based Facility;
- Distinct Part Unit;
- or files a consolidated cost report,

then the organization must provide the name and Medicare identification number of their parent provider.
> **Note:** The final determination as to whether an entity is truly a Provider Based Facility will be made by HCFA prior to completion of the enrollment process.

In addition to the parent provider relationship described above, the organization must identify how many Provider Based Facilities, Distinct Part Units, Branches, or Multi-campus sites the organization is responsible for. For each of those locations identified, the Practice Location(s) section of this application must be completed.

If applicant receives payment from Medicare or any other federal health care agency for any services rendered by a contractor, when permitted by Medicare or other federal health care program requirements, the contractor must complete and sign the HCFA Form 855R (Individual Reassignment of Benefits Application).

C. Physician and Non-Physician Practitioner Groups Only

Complete all items in this section. Furnish the group's legal business name. This should be the legal name used in reporting to the IRS. Furnish the group's primary specialty (the primary specialty of the majority of the group's members). Designation of a secondary specialty is optional. All group members who the group will be billing the Medicare or other federal health care program in their behalf, must be individually enrolled in the given Medicare or other federal health care program.

> **Note:** The group's members must be enrolled within the same federal health care program as the group enrollment. Otherwise, the group member must enroll separately as an individual in the group's federal health care program prior to becoming a member of that group practice.

Each group member must complete and sign the HCFA Form 855R (Individual Reassignment of Benefits Application).

> **Note: PARTNERSHIPS:** When completing this section, provide legal business name of partnership, date partnership was incorporated, and the State where the partnership is incorporated. Place "n/a" in the specialty block.

D. All Applicants

Provide applicant's mailing address. This is where the applicant can receive correspondence and bulletins from Medicare or other federal health care program contractors. This address may be the applicant's home address or a Post Office Box. Applicant must supply fax number and e-mail address if available. If applicable, provide applicant's previously assigned Medicare Identification Number(s) and the name(s) of the Carrier and/or Fiscal Intermediary to which applicant most recently submitted bills using this number. If applicable, provide applicant's most recent Medicaid number and the State in which it was issued. Applicant must provide his/her social security number and when applicable, his/her employer identification number(s).

> **Note:** All applicants **must** provide either their social security number and/or, when applicable, their employer identification number (EIN). **If applicant uses more than one EIN, list all, starting with the EIN(s) currently used or to be used for tax reporting purposes relating to this application. Attach a copy of IRS Form CP 575 to verify the applicant's EIN.**

Applicant must answer all questions related to criminal activity. Answering "yes" to any of these questions will not automatically deny enrollment into Medicare or other federal health care programs. For purposes of these questions related to criminal activity, an "immediate family member" of the applicant is defined as:
- a husband or wife;
- the natural or adoptive parent, child or sibling;
- the stepparent, stepchild, stepbrother or stepsister;
- the father, mother, daughter, son, brother or sister;
- parent-in-law, brother-in-law or sister-in-law;
- the grandparent or grandchild; and
- the spouse of a grandparent or grandchild.

For purposes of these questions related to criminal activity, "member of household" with respect to the applicant is defined as any individual sharing a common abode as part of a single family unit with the applicant, including domestic employees and others who live together as a family unit, but not including a roomer or boarder.

Indicate whether the applicant (under the name of the applicant shown on this application or any other name) has any outstanding overpayments with Medicare, Medicaid or any other federal program. If the applicant has an outstanding overpayment, furnish the name of the federal program where the overpayment exists. If this outstanding overpayment is in a name other than the name identified in the Applicant Identification section, furnish the other name in the space provided.

2. Professional and Business License, Certification, and Registration Information

All applicants are required to furnish information on all Federal, State and local (city/county) professional and business licenses, certifications and/or registrations required to practice as applicant's provider/supplier type in applicant's (e.g. State medical license for physician, State certification and/or registration for Nurses, Federal DEA number, Business Occupancy License, local business license, etc.). The local Medicare or other federal health care contractor will supply specific credentialing requirements for applicant's provider/supplier type upon request.

Notarized or "certified true" copies of the above information are optional, but will speed the processing of this application.

> **Notarized:** A notarized copy of an original document that will have a stamp which states "Official Seal" along with the name and signature of the notary public, State, County, and the date the notary's commission expires.

> **Certified True:** This is a copy of the original document obtained from where it originated or is stored, and it has a raised seal which identifies the State and County in which it originated or is stored.

In lieu of copies of the above requested documents, the applicant may submit a notarized or "certified true" Certificate of Good Standing from the applicant's State licensing/certification board or other medical association. This certificate cannot be more than 30 days old.

Non-physician practitioners who must meet Medicare or other federal health care program requirements for professional experience should submit evidence of practice and the dates of employment.

If applicant's enrollment requires a State survey and/or certification, the applicant is required to forward copies of State survey and/or certification documents to the Medicare or other federal health care contractor once they are received from the State agency or Regional Medicare Office.

> **Note:** Temporary licenses are acceptable submissions with this application. However, once received, a copy of the applicant's permanent license must be forwarded to the Medicare or other federal health care program contractor within 30 days of receipt.

If applicant's State licensure is dependent upon State survey and/or certification, check applicable box and furnish information on all other required licensing information.

> **Note:** A business license is required for each practice location.

If applicant had a previously revoked or suspended license, certification, or registration reinstated, attach a copy of the reinstatement notice(s) with this application, if applicable.

3. Professional School Information (Individuals Only)

If applicable, supply information about the educational institution from which applicant received medical, professional, or related degree or training as required by applicant's State. Enclose copies of diploma, degree or evidence of qualifying course work.

Non-physician practitioners who must meet HCFA or other federal health care program requirements for education must provide documentation of courses or degrees taken that satisfy Medicare or other federal health care program requirements. Contact the local Medicare or other federal health care program representative for requirements needed for applicant's provider/supplier type.

4. Board Certification

If applicant is Board Certified, furnish requested information for each Board Certification obtained by the applicant.

5. Exclusion/Sanction Information

Supply all requested information. If applicable, attach copy(s) of any official documentation related to the adverse legal action identified, including reinstatement notices. If applicant has not had any adverse legal actions, check the "none of these" box.

6. Practice Location(s)

Provide all information requested for each location where applicant will render services to Medicare or other federal health care program beneficiaries.

Individual practitioners should include all hospitals and/or other health care facilities where they render service or have privileges to treat patients. Individual practitioners who only render services in the patient's home (house calls) should supply his/her home address in this section. If individual practitioners render services in retirement or assisted living communities, complete this section using the names and addresses of these communities.

Hospitals must list all off-site clinics, distinct part units, and provider based facilities (e.g., skilled nursing facility, rural health clinic, etc.) and multi-campus sites.

Home health agencies and hospices must list all branches.

> **Note:** Listing the facilities, clinics, units, and multi-campus sites controlled by a hospital or other entity does not automatically enroll them in the Medicare or other federal health program. The HCFA Form 855 (General Enrollment Application) must also be completed for each of these entities.

Post Office boxes and drop boxes are **not** acceptable as practice location addresses. The phone number must be a number where patients and/or customers can reach the applicant to ask questions or register complaints.

Furnish the "Pay To" address for payment of services rendered at this practice location. Payments will be made in the legal business name that the individual, organization, or group/partnership uses to report to the IRS, as reported in Section 1 of this application. In most circumstances, payment will be made in the name of the individual who furnished the service unless a valid Reassignment of Benefits Statement has been completed. The "Pay To" address may be a Post Office box.

Furnish the name and social security number of the primary managing/directing employee of this practice location.

If applicable, provide the CLIA number or FDA certification number associated with each piece of equipment at each practice location and submit a copy of the most current certification.

6. Practice Location(s) (continued)

Indicate whether patient records are kept on the premises. If not, supply the name of the storage facility/location and the physical address where the records are maintained. Post Office boxes and drop boxes are **not** acceptable as the physical address where patient records are maintained.

7. Prior Practice Information

FOR MEDICARE ENROLLMENT ONLY

If applicant has previously billed Medicare or Medicaid, supply requested information about the prior practice. Indicate whether applicant was a participating or non-participating provider/supplier in the prior practice.

8. Ownership Information

Complete this section for all individuals and/or entities who have an ownership or control interest in the applicant's business/entity. If owner is an individual, complete owner name, social security number and employer identification number. If applicant is owned by another entity, complete legal business name and employer identification number of the owning entity as well as the name(s) and social security number of each owner of that entity. Entities with ownership interest must provide their legal business name(s).

A person or entity with an ownership or control interest is one that:

- has an ownership interest totaling 5% or more in the provider/supplier;

- has a direct, indirect, or combination of direct and indirect ownership interest equal to 5% or more in the provider/supplier, where the amount of an indirect ownership interest is determined by multiplying the percentages of ownership in each entity (for example, if A owns 10 % of the stock in a corporation that owns 80% of the provider/supplier, A's interest equates to an 8% indirect ownership interest in the provider/supplier and must be reported);

- owns an interest of 5% or more in any mortgage, deed of trust, note or other obligation secured by the provider/supplier if that interest equals at least 5% of the value of the property or assets of the provider/supplier;

- is an officer or director of a provider/supplier that is organized as a corporation; and/or

- is a partner in a provider/supplier that is organized as a partnership.

Supply all requested information about the owner's past and present billing relationships with Medicare. Furnish past history for the last 10 years. If data is not known or is incomplete, check the appropriate box.

Supply all requested adverse legal action information about the owner(s). If applicable, attach copy(s) of any official documentation related to the adverse legal action identified, including reinstatement notices. If none of the owner(s) has had any adverse legal actions, check the "none of these" box.

Attach a copy of the applicant's IRS Form CP 575 pertaining to this business. The IRS Form CP 575 will be used to verify the employer identification number (EIN).

In lieu of the IRS Form CP 575, the applicant may use any official correspondence, such as the quarterly tax payment coupon, from the IRS showing the name of the entity as shown on this application and the EIN.

9. Managing/Directing Employees

Complete this section for all managing and/or directing employees, employed by the applicant. This section should include, but is not limited to, general manager(s), business manager(s), administrator(s), director(s), or other individuals who exercise operational or managerial control over the provider/supplier, or who directly or indirectly conduct the applicant's day-to-day operations.

Note: This section **is not** to be completed with information about billing agency or management service organization employees. If applicant uses a billing agency or management service organization, complete the appropriate section of this application.

Note: Non-profit organizations should complete this section with information about the members on the Board of Directors and the managing and/or directing employees and submit a copy of the 501(C)(3) approval notification from the IRS.

Note: For large business organizations, furnish only the top 20 compensated managing and/or directing personnel. Social security numbers <u>must</u> be provided for all persons listed in this section.

Applicant must include all managing and/or directing employees for each practice location. Organizations must also complete this section for all corporate officers. Include the name(s) and address(es) of all practice location(s) where this employee manages and/or directs.

Supply all requested information about the managing and/or directing employee's past and present billing relationships with Medicare or other federal health care programs.

Supply all requested information about other entities this managing and/or directing employee managed or directed that previously billed or are presently billing the Medicare or other federal health care programs. Furnish past history for the last 10 years. If data is not known or is incomplete, check the box indicating this.

Supply all requested information about other entities this managing and/or directing employee had ownership interest in that previously billed or are presently billing the Medicare or other federal health care programs. Furnish past history for the last 10 years. If data is not known or is incomplete, check the appropriate box.

Supply all requested adverse legal information about the managing/directing employee(s). If applicable, attach copy(s) of any official documentation related to the adverse legal action identified, including reinstatement notices. If none of the managing/directing employee(s) has had any adverse legal actions, check the "none of these" box.

10. Parent/Joint Venture or Subsidiary Information

If applicant is a subsidiary (wholly or partially owned by another organization or business), or a joint venture (equally owned by another individual(s), organization(s) or business(s)), complete all information requested in this section <u>about the parent company or joint venture</u>. Attach a copy of the parent company's or other owner's IRS Form CP 575 pertaining to this business.

11. Chain Organization Information

When applicable, this section to be completed by Medicare Part A Institutional provider/suppliers ONLY. This includes all institutional chain provider/suppliers that bill fiscal intermediaries (e.g., Home Health Agencies and Skilled Nursing Facilities).

If applicant is in a chain organization, check appropriate action block for this chain, then supply all information requested <u>about the chain home office</u>.

12. Contractor Information (Business Organizations)

This section is to be completed with information about all business organizations that the applicant contracts with that:

- provide medical or diagnostic services or medical supplies for which the cost or value is $10,000 or more in a 12 month period; OR

- will reassign benefits to the applicant, regardless of annual cost or value of medical or diagnostic services or medical supplies provided.

Provide all requested information about the contractor's past and present billing relationships with Medicare or Medicaid.

Supply all requested adverse legal action information about the contractor(s). If applicable, attach copy(s) of any official documentation related to the adverse legal action identified, including reinstatement notices. If none of the contractor(s) has had any adverse legal actions, check the "none of these" box.

If a <u>business or group contractor</u> will be reassigning Medicare or other federal health care program benefits to the applicant, an authorized representative of the <u>business or group contractor</u> must complete and sign the Reassignment of Benefits section of <u>this application</u>. See instructions below for additional reassignment of benefits information.

> **Note:** <u>Individuals</u> with whom the applicant contracts with to do business <u>and</u> who will reassign benefits to the applicant must complete the **HCFA Form 855R** (Individual Reassignment of Benefits Application).

If a currently enrolled provider/supplier is obtaining the services of a new contractor that will be reassigning its benefits, complete only the Application Identification section, the Contractor Information section and the Reassignment of Benefits Statement.

13. Reassignment of Benefits Statement

In general, Medicare and other federal health care programs make payment only to the beneficiary or the individual or entity that directly provides the service.

Reassigned benefits must be within the same federal health care program (e.g., Medicare to Medicare, CHAMPUS to CHAMPUS, etc.).

If the applicant receives payment on behalf of other business organizations for services provided, the other business organization must complete and sign the Reassignment of Benefits Statement. Failure to do so will cause a delay in processing the application and limit the Medicare or other federal

health care program contractor's ability to make payment.

This section must be signed by an Authorized Representative of the entity reassigning its benefits to this applicant.

The reassignee is permitted by Federal law to reassign Medicare benefits to an employer, the facility where the service is rendered, a health care delivery system, or agent. For further information on Federal requirements on reassignment of benefits the applicant should contact the local Medicare or other federal health care program contractor before signing the application.

The Legal Business Name of the applicant must be the same as the Legal Business Name of the applicant identified in Section 1 of this application.

Individual practitioners, including individual contractors and group members, who reassign Medicare or other federal health care program benefits to this applicant must complete the HCFA Form 855R. Individual practitioners who are contracted by the applicant, but do not reassign their benefits to the applicant do not need to complete the HCFA Form 855R.

14. Billing Agency/Management Service Organization Address

A Billing Agency is a company contracted by the applicant to furnish all claims processing functions for the applicant's practice.

A Management Service Organization is a company contracted by the applicant to furnish some or all administrative, clerical and claims processing functions of the applicant's practice.

If the applicant currently uses or will be using a billing agency and/or management service organization to submit bills, complete all requested information and attach a current copy of the signed contract between the applicant and the billing agency or management service organization.

> **Note:** If applicant uses a billing agency and/ or management service organization but no written contract exists between applicant and billing agency and/or management service organization, a contract must be written and furnished with this application.

Any change in the contract between the applicant and the billing agency and/or management service organization <u>must</u> be reported to the Medicare or other federal health care program contractor within 30 calendar days of said change.

15. Electronic Claims Submission Information

If applicant plans to submit bills electronically, or would like information about electronic billing, supply a contact name and phone number. The Medicare or other federal health care program contractor will be in contact with further instructions about qualifying for electronic billing submissions.

> **Note:** Electronic Funds Transfer can only be made into an account controlled exclusively by the applicant.

16. Surety Bond Information

Complete all requested information.

Annual surety bond renewals must be reported to the Medicare or other federal health care program contractor using HCFA Form 855C (Change of Information Form).

16. Surety Bond Information (continued)

An original copy of the surety bond must be submitted with this application. Failure to submit a copy of the surety bond will prevent the processing of this application. In addition, the applicant must obtain and submit a certified copy of the agent's Power of Attorney with this application, if the bond is issued by an agent.

17. Contact Person

Provide the full name and telephone number of an individual who can be reached to answer questions regarding the information furnished in this application.

18. Certification Statement

This statement includes the minimum standards to which the applicant must adhere to be enrolled in Medicare or other federal health care programs. Read these statements carefully.

By signing the Certification Statement, the applicant agrees to adhere to all the conditions listed and is aware that the applicant may be denied entry to or revoked from the program if any conditions are violated. The Certification Statement must contain an original signature. Faxed or photocopied signatures will not be accepted.

> **Note:** If applicant is applying as an individual or sole proprietor, **applicant** must sign and date the Certification Statement. If applicant is applying as an organization or as a group practice, **an authorized representative of the organization/group practice** must sign the Certification Statement. If applicant has more than one authorized representative, furnish the names and signatures of those authorized representatives who will be directly involved with the Medicare or other federal health care contractors.

Attachment 1   Ambulance Service Suppliers

This attachment is to be completed by the applicant for each ambulance service company being enrolled in the Medicare or other federal health care program.

1. State License Information

If applicant is currently State licensed and certified to operate as an ambulance service supplier, complete this section and attach copy(s) of all State licenses and documents.

A copy of applicant's current license or certificate must be attached to this form. The effective date and expiration date must be stated on the license or certificate. Claims will be paid based on these dates. The applicant must provide this office with a copy of the renewal license in order to receive payment after the expiration date.

2. Description of Vehicle(s)

Applicant must identify the type (e.g., automobile, aircraft, boat) of each vehicle, and furnish year, make, model, and vehicle identification number.

The applicant's vehicle(s) must be specially designed and equipped for transporting the sick or injured. It must have customary patient care equipment including, but not limited to, a stretcher, clean linens, first aid supplies and oxygen equipment, and it must have all other safety and lifesaving equipment as required by State and local authorities. If the ambulance will supply Advanced Life Support services, list all the necessary equipment and provide documentation of certification from the authorized licensing and regulation agency for applicant's area of operation.

Vehicles must be regularly inspected and recertified according to applicable State and local licensure laws. Evidence of recertification must be submitted to the Medicare or other federal health care program contractor on an ongoing basis, as required by State or local law.

   Note: Air Ambulance

To qualify for air ambulance, the following is required:

- a written statement that gives the name and address of the facility where the aircraft is hangared signed by the President, Chief Executive Officer, or Chief Operating Officer of the airport; and

- proof that the air ambulance applicant or its leasing company possess a valid charter flight license (FAA 135 Certificate) for the aircraft being used as an air ambulance. If the air medical transportation company owns the aircraft, the owner's name on the FAA 135 Certificate must be the same as the applicant's name on this enrollment application. If the air medical transportation company leases the aircraft, a copy of the lease agreement must accompany this enrollment application. The name of the company leasing the aircraft must be the same as the applicant's name on this enrollment application.

3. Qualification of Crew

The ambulance crew must consist of at least two members. Those crew members charged with the care or handling of the patient must include one individual with adequate first aid training, (i.e., training at least equivalent to that provided by the basic and advanced Red Cross first aid courses). If the ambulance crew will provide ALS services, they must list their ALS training courses.

Training "equivalent" to the basic and advanced Red Cross first aid courses include ambulance service training and experience acquired in military service and/or successful completion by the individual of a comparable first aid course furnished by or under the sponsorship of State or local authorities, an educational institution, a fire department, a hospital, a professional organization, or other such qualified organization.

Applicant must enclose a certificate(s) showing that crew members have successfully completed the required first aid training, or give a description of the equivalent military training, where and when it was received. Crew must continue to pursue and complete continuing education requirements in accordance with State and local licensure laws. Evidence of recertification must be submitted to the Medicare or other federal health care program contractor on an ongoing basis, as required by State and local law.

4. Billing Method

FOR MEDICARE ENROLLMENT ONLY

Answer all applicable questions regarding billing methods. Supply the name of the Medical Director and the geographic area the applicant services.

   Note: Paramedic Intercept Services:

- A basic life support (BLS) ambulance supplier may arrange with a paramedic/Emergency Medical Technician (EMT) organization or another advanced life support (ALS) ambulance supplier to provide the advanced life support services while it provides for the transportation component. The BLS would bill for the ALS services and make arrangement to pay the organization providing the ALS services. As an alternative, the BLS could arrange for the organization providing the ALS to be its billing agent.

- If this alternate arrangement exists, applicant must complete the Billing Agency/Management Service Organization and Reassignment of Benefits section and submit a copy of the signed contract.

Check the appropriate box indicating if applicant bills for nautical miles or statute miles.

If applicant is not enrolling in the Medicare program skip this section.

5. Exclusion/Sanction Information

Supply all requested adverse legal action information about the ambulance crew member(s). If applicable, attach copy(s) of any official documentation related to the adverse legal action identified, including reinstatement notices. If none of the ambulance crew members has had any adverse legal actions, check the appropriate box and skip this section.

Attachment 2   Independent Diagnostic Testing Facilities (IDTFs)

Formerly known as Independent Physiological Laboratories.

This attachment is to be completed by the applicant for each Independent Diagnostic Testing Facility being enrolled in the Medicare or other federal health care program.

Definition:

Independent Diagnostic Testing Facility (IDTF): An entity independent of a hospital or physician's office in which diagnostic tests are performed by licensed, certified non-physician personnel under appropriate physician supervision (e.g., free standing cardiac catherization facility, imaging center).

> **Note:** A cardiac catherization facility which is a physician's office is not an IDTF. The term "free standing" means that the cardiac catherization facility, whether office or IDTF, is independent of a hospital.

1. Identification of Practice Location

Indicate whether this practice location is operating as a mobile unit. If so, provide vehicle identification number and expiration date of vehicle license. If operating mobile units, the vehicles must be regularly inspected and recertified according to State and local licensure laws. Evidence of recertification must be submitted to the Medicare or other federal health care program contractor on an ongoing basis, as required by State and local law.

Identify practice location of IDTF for which this attachment is being completed. If this is a mobile unit, furnish the address where the vehicle is stored.

If applicable, complete all information concerning applicant's practice location.

2. Identification of Supervising/Directing Physician(s)

The information in this section is required only if applicant's State requires that a supervising physician be associated with all IDTFs. Supervising physicians must perform their duties as described by State requirements. Each supervising/directing physician is required to be enrolled as an individual practitioner in Medicare or other federal health care program for which the applicant is applying.

3. Service Performance

List all Current Procedural Terminology, Version 4 (CPT-4) and HCFA Common Procedure Coding System (HCPCS) codes this IDTF or its contractors intend to perform, supervise, interpret, or bill. Describe the setting where the service will be rendered, and identify each physician who will be performing, supervising, and/or interpreting the test results.

4. Referral Records

Explain how referral records, physician's written order and the name of the technician who rendered the service are maintained.

5. Supervising/Directing Physician Exclusion/Sanction Information

Supply all requested adverse legal action information about the supervising/directing physician(s). If applicable, attach copy(s) of any official documentation related to the adverse legal action identified, including reinstatement notices. If none of the supervising/directing physician(s) has had any adverse legal actions, check the "none of these" box.

6. Signature of Supervising/Directing Physician(s)

Each supervising/directing physician identified in Section 2 of this attachment must sign this attachment.

Attachment 3   Home Health Agencies (HHAs)

This attachment is to be completed by all Home Health Agencies for enrollment in the Medicare or other federal health care program.

This attachment must be completed with information about other related business interests in which the HHA itself has a 5% or more ownership interest in or control of the other related business.

In addition, each owner listed in the Ownership Information section **and** each managing/directing employee listed in the Managing/Directing Employee section who has a 5% or more ownership interest in or controls the other related businesses (as defined below) must complete this attachment.

Copy and submit a separate Attachment 3 for the HHA, each owner and each managing/directing employee, as applicable.

—

Definitions:

Related to the Provider: Related to the provider (HHA) means that the provider (HHA), to a significant extent, is associated or affiliated with or has control of or is controlled by an organization furnishing services, facilities, or supplies to the provider.

Common Ownership: Common ownership exists if an individual or individuals possess significant ownership or equity in the provider (HHA) **and** the institution or organization serving the provider (HHA).

Control Interest: Control exists if an owner of the HHA has the power, directly or indirectly, to significantly influence or direct the actions or policies of an organization or institution furnishing services, facilities, or supplies to the provider (HHA).

1. Other Related Business Interests

The HHA itself and all owners and managing/directing employees of the enrolling Home Health Agency are required to furnish identifying information about all other related businesses in which they have a 5% or more ownership in and/or control interest.

In general, businesses than furnish services, facilities, and supplies to the provider (HHA) that are related to the provider (HHA) by common ownership or control interest are to be listed in this attachment.

Supply all requested information about the related businesses.

For purposes of this application, the definition of related businesses as found in 42 CFR § 413.17 which concerns ownership and control, and is limited to businesses who actually do business with the HHA being enrolled will be used. These rules apply regardless of that business' relationship to Medicare, Medicaid or any other health care program, industry, or business.

Examples of related businesses:

- if an HHA, or the owner, or the managing/directing employee owns a small retail store that has no business dealings with the HHA, the store is not considered to be a related business;

- a consulting firm owned by the HHA, one of the HHA owners, or one of the HHA managing/directing employees, which provides management services to the HHA would be considered a related business; and

- a retail business owned by the HHA, one of the HHA owners, or one of the HHA managing/directing employees, which provides supplies to the HHA would be considered a related business.

Identify the type of business in which the related business is engaged (e.g., durable medical equipment company, consulting firm).

Identify the relationship of the related business to the HHA (e.g., affiliate, joint venture, supplier).

According to the Paperwork Reduction Act of 1995, no persons are required to respond to a collection of information unless it displays a valid OMB control number. The valid OMB control number for this information collection is 0938-0685. The time required to complete this information collection is estimated at 1 ½ - 3 hours per response, including the time to review instructions, search existing data resources, gather the data needed, and complete and review the information collection. If you have any comments concerning the accuracy of the time estimate(s) or suggestions for improving this form, please write to: HCFA, P.O. Box 26684, Baltimore, Maryland 21207 and to the Office of Information and Regulatory Affairs, Office of Management and Budget, Washington, D.C. 20503.

MEDICARE/FEDERAL HEALTH CARE PROVIDER/SUPPLIER ENROLLMENT APPLICATION
General Application

PLEASE CHECK APPLICABLE BOX

Type of Business: ☐ Individual ☐ Corporation ☐ Partnership ☐ Other (specify) _____

Applicant   PLEASE CHECK APPLICABLE BOX
Enrolling As: ☐ Individual ☐ Sole Proprietor ☐ Organization ☐ Group ☐ Mass Immunization Biller Only

Check the appropriate box listed below if applicant is completing this application for enrollment in a federal health care program other than Medicare. (Check only one program box.)   ☐ State Medicaid   ☐ CHAMPUS   ☐ Indian Health Service
   ☐ Railroad Retirement Board   ☐ Public Health Service   ☐ CHAMPVA   ☐ Other (specify) _____

PLEASE CHECK APPLICABLE BOX

Application For: ☐ Initial Enrollment   ☐ Recertification   ☐ Change of Ownership (CHOW)
   ☐ Enrollment of Additional Location(s)   ☐ Change of Information

MEDICARE APPLICANTS ONLY:
Where will applicant be submitting billings? ☐ Fiscal Intermediary ☐ Carrier ☐ Both (OR) ☐ Regional Home Health Intermediary
If fiscal intermediary is checked, furnish name of applicant's preferred fiscal intermediary. _____

Is the applicant currently enrolled in another federal health care program? ☐ YES ☐ NO
IF YES, check all the appropriate federal programs listed below.
   ☐ Medicare   ☐ State Medicaid   ☐ CHAMPUS   ☐ Indian Health Service
   ☐ Railroad Retirement Board   ☐ Public Health Service   ☐ CHAMPVA   ☐ Other (specify) _____

1. Applicant Identification

A. Individuals ONLY
Check here ☐ only if this entire section does not apply to the applicant.

Name:	First	Middle	Last	Jr., Sr., etc,	M.D., D.O., etc.

Other Name:	First	Middle	Last	Jr., Sr., etc.	M.D., D.O., etc.

Residency Status (if applicable)   ☐ resident   ☐ intern
Name of Facility Where Resident or Intern:

_____

Are services rendered in the above setting part of the applicant's requirements for graduation from a formal residency program? ☐ YES ☐ NO
Primary Specialty (e.g. pathology, cardiology, nurse practitioner, etc.) (required)   Secondary Specialty (if applicable)

Gender (optional)   ☐ male   ☐ female

Race/Ethnicity (optional) ☐ Asian or Asian American or Pacific Islander   ☐ Hispanic   ☐ Black (not Hispanic) or African-American   ☐ North American Indian or Alaska Native   ☐ White (not Hispanic)

Date of Birth (MM/DD/YYYY)	County of Birth	State of Birth	Country of Birth

B. Organizations ONLY
Check here ☐ only if this entire section does not apply to the applicant.

1. Legal Business Name	Fiscal Year End Date (MM/DD)	Incorporation Date (if applicable) (MM/DD/YYYY)

Type of Facility (e.g., hospital, nursing home, clinical laboratory, roster biller, etc.)	☐ Accredited ☐ Non-Accredited

State Where Incorporated:	Date Business Established at This Location (MM/DD/YYYY)	All other States in which applicant does business:

2. Is this a organization a Provider Based Facility? ☐ Yes ☐ No   Is this organization a Distinct Part Unit? ☐ Yes ☐ No
Does this organization file a consolidated cost report under another Medicare provider's number? ☐ Yes ☐ No
IF YES to any of the above three questions, furnish name of parent provider.   Parent Medicare Provider Number

3. Does this organization operate other affiliated units, off-site clinics, or have multi-campus sites or branches? ☐ Yes ☐ No
If Yes, how many of each? _____ other affiliated units _____ off-site clinics _____ multi-campus sites _____ branches
Complete the Practice Location(s) section for each unit, clinic, site, and/or branch operated.

1. Applicant Identification (continued)

C. Physician and Non-Physician Practitioner Groups ONLY (For each group member, complete HCFA Form 855R.)

Check here ☐ only if this entire section does not apply to the applicant.

Legal Business Name	Incorporation Date (if applicable) (MM/DD/YYYY)	State Where Incorporated
Group's Primary Specialty (required)	Group's Secondary Specialty (if applicable)	

D. All Applicants

1. Mailing Address Line 1

Mailing Address Line 2

City	County	State	ZIP Code + 4
Telephone Number	Fax Number		E-mail Address
Employer Identification Number (if applicable)	Social Security Number (if applicable)		Medicare Identification Number(s) (if applicable)

2. Does applicant now have or has applicant ever had a Medicare or Medicaid provider number in this or any other State?

☐ Yes ☐ No   IF YES, supply all current and prior information requested below.

Current Carrier Name (if applicable)	Current Intermediary Name (if applicable)	Current Medicaid Number/State (if applicable)
Prior Carrier Name (if applicable)	Prior Intermediary Name (if applicable)	Prior Medicaid Number/State (if applicable)
Current CLIA Number (if applicable)	Prior CLIA Number (if applicable)	

3. Has applicant ever been convicted of any health care related crime?   ☐ Yes ☐ No

Has applicant ever been convicted of a felony under Federal or State law?   ☐ Yes ☐ No

4. Has any family and/or household member(s) of the applicant who has ownership or control interest in the enrolling business or entity ever been convicted, assessed, or excluded from the Medicare program due to fraud, obstruction of an investigation, or a controlled substance violation?

☐ Yes ☐ No   IF YES, furnish name and relationship of relative/household member(s) below.

Name: First	Middle	Last	Jr., Sr., etc,	Relationship

5. Does the applicant, under any name or business identity, have any outstanding overpayments with Medicare, Medicaid or any other federal program?

☐ Yes ☐ No   IF YES, under what federal program? _____

IF YES, under what name? _____

2. Professional and Business License/Certification/Registration Information

Attach a copy(s) of each required Federal, State, and/or local city/county business and/or professional license, certification and/or registration. Notarized or "certified true" copies are optional but will speed the processing of this application.

Check here ☐ if applicant's State licensure is pending upon completion of State survey and/or certification.

Has applicant ever had any Federal, State, and/or local city/county business and/or professional business license, certification and/or registration revoked or suspended?   ☐ Yes ☐ No

IF YES, explain below and attach copy(s) of reinstatement letter(s) if applicable.

_____

_____

3. Professional School Information (Individuals only)

Check here ☐ only if this entire section does not apply to the applicant.

Attach a copy of each degree or certificate. Notarized or "certified true" copies are optional but will speed the processing of this application.

School Name	Graduation Year (YYYY)
City	State	Country

4. Board Certification

Check here ☐ only if this entire section does not apply to the applicant.

If applicant is Board Certified in his/her primary specialty complete the following information.

If applicant is Board Certified in more than one specialty, copy this section and complete the following information for each.

Certification Board Name

Certification Number	Effective Date (MM/DD/YYYY)	Expiration Date (MM/DD/YYYY)

5. Exclusion/Sanction Information

Check if the applicant has **ever** had any of the following adverse legal actions imposed by the Medicare, Medicaid, or any other federal agency or program. For each box checked, include the date the adverse legal action was imposed.

Check all that apply or the "none of these" box. Attach copy of adverse legal action notification.

1.
☐ Administrative Sanction(s) _____
☐ Program exclusion(s) _____
☐ Suspension of payment(s) _____
☐ Civil monetary penalty(s) _____
☐ Assessment(s) _____
☐ Program Debarment(s) _____

2. Health Care Related:
☐ Criminal fine(s) _____
☐ Restitution order(s) _____
☐ Pending civil judgment(s) _____
☐ Pending criminal judgment(s) _____
☐ Judgment(s) pending under the False Claims Act _____

3. ☐ None of these
_____
_____

D. Does the applicant have any outstanding criminal fines? ☐ Yes ☐ No   restitution orders? ☐ Yes ☐ No

6. Practice Location(s)

Check here ☐ if deleting this practice location.

A. How many practice locations does applicant utilize? _____ For each additional practice location, copy and complete this section.

B. "Doing Business As" name for this location	Medicare Identification Number for this location (if applicable)

Business Street Address Line 1

Business Street Address Line 2

City	County	State	ZIP Code + 4

Telephone Number	Fax Number	E-mail Address

Is this location an ☐ off site clinic? ☐ distinct part unit? ☐ multi-campus site? ☐ branch?
☐ a location that files a consolidated cost report? ☐ provider based facility? ☐ or none of these?

Date applicant began practicing at this location? (MM/DD/YYYY)	If applicable, date applicant ceased practicing at this location? (MM/DD/YYYY)

Check whether the applicant owns or leases this practice location? ☐ Own ☐ Lease

C. "Pay To" address for this practice location. Check here ☐ and skip to section 6D if same as practice location in section 6B.

Check here ☐ if applicant wants all practice location payments listed in this application sent to address furnished in Section 6C.

Mailing Address Line 1

Mailing Address Line 2

City	State	ZIP Code + 4	Telephone Number

D. Name of managing/directing employee for this location?	First	Middle	Last	Social Security Number

E. CLIA Number for this location (if applicable)	FDA Mammography Certification Number(s) for this location (if applicable)

F. Are all patient records stored at this practice location? ☐ Yes ☐ No   IF NO, supply storage location below.

Name of Storage Facility/Location	Telephone Number	Fax Number

Street Address Line 1

Street Address Line 2

City	State	ZIP Code + 4

7. Prior Practice Information

Check here ☐ only if this entire section does not apply to the applicant.

If applicant has previously billed the Medicare or Medicaid programs, furnish requested prior practice information below.
For each additional prior practice, copy and complete this section.

Type of Practice	Status	☐ Inactive	IF INACTIVE, supply date of termination (MM/DD/YYYY)
		☐ Active	_____

Legal Business Name

Doing Business As Name

Medicare Identification Number(s)	Medicaid Number/State	Telephone Number

Business Street Address Line 1

Business Street Address Line 2

City	State	ZIP Code + 4

Was applicant a ☐ participating or ☐ non-participating provider/supplier in this prior practice?

8. Ownership Information

Check here ☐ if deleting this owner's association with this entity.

Effective date of deletion? _____ (MM/DD/YYYY)

How many owners have 5 percent or more ownership interest in this entity?_____ (maximum of 20)

For each owner, complete this section. If more than one owner, copy and complete this section for each.

All applicants must submit a copy of the entity's IRS Form CP 575.

A. Identifying Information

Owner Name: First	Middle	Last	Jr., Sr., etc.	M.D., D.O., etc.

Other Name: First	Middle	Last	Jr., Sr., etc.	M.D., D.O., etc.

Date of Birth (MM/DD/YYYY)	County of Birth	State of Birth	Country of Birth

Legal Business Name

"Doing Business As" Name	Effective Date of Ownership (MM/DD/YYYY)

Social Security Number	Employer Identification Number	Medicare Identification Number (if applicable)

B. Does this owner now have or has this owner ever had a Medicare or Medicaid provider number in this or any other State?

☐ Yes ☐ No   IF YES, supply all current and prior information requested below.

Current Carrier Name (if applicable)	Current Fiscal Intermediary Name (if applicable)	Current Medicaid Number/State (if applicable)
Prior Carrier Name (if applicable)	Prior Fiscal Intermediary Name (if applicable)	Prior Medicaid Number/State (if applicable)

C. Has this owner ever managed or directed other organizations that have billed or are currently billing Medicare for services?

☐ Yes ☐ No   IF YES, how many? _____

Copy and complete the following for each organization this owner managed or directed in the last 10 years.

If this list is incomplete, check here ☐ indicating that some information for the last 10 years is missing.

Organization's Legal Business Name

Employer Identification Number	Medicare Identification Number	Date Associated FROM — TO (MM/DD/YYYY)
Current Carrier Name (if applicable)	Current Fiscal Intermediary Name (if applicable)	Current Medicaid Number/State (if applicable)
Prior Carrier Name (if applicable)	Prior Fiscal Intermediary Name (if applicable)	Prior Medicaid Number/State (if applicable)

8. Ownership Information (continued)

D. Has this owner ever had ownership in other organizations that have billed or are currently billing Medicare for services?

☐ Yes   ☐ No   IF YES, how many? _____

Copy and complete the following for each organization this owner has had ownership in during the last 10 years.

If this list is incomplete, check here ☐ indicating that some information for the last 10 years is missing.

Organization's Legal Business Name

Employer Identification Number	Medicare Identification Number	Date Associated FROM — TO (MM/DD/YYYY)
Current Carrier Name (if applicable)	Current Fiscal Intermediary Name (if applicable)	Current Medicaid Number/State (if applicable)
Prior Carrier Name (if applicable)	Prior Fiscal Intermediary Name (if applicable)	Prior Medicaid Number/State (if applicable)

E. Check if this owner has <u>ever</u> had any of the following adverse legal actions imposed by the Medicare, Medicaid, or any other federal agency or program. For each box checked, include the date the adverse legal action was imposed.

Check all that apply or the "none of these" box. Attach copy of adverse legal action notification.

1.
☐ Administrative Sanction(s) _____
☐ Program exclusion(s) _____
☐ Suspension of payment(s) _____
☐ Civil monetary penalty(s) _____
☐ Assessment(s) _____
☐ Program Debarment(s) _____

2. Health Care Related:
☐ Criminal fine(s) _____
☐ Restitution order(s) _____
☐ Pending civil judgment(s) _____
☐ Pending criminal judgment(s) _____
☐ Judgment(s) pending under the False Claims Act _____

3. ☐ None of these

4. Does this owner have any outstanding criminal fines? ☐ Yes ☐ No   restitution orders? ☐ Yes ☐ No

F. Has this owner ever been convicted of any health care related crime? ☐ Yes ☐ No

   Has this owner ever been convicted of a felony under Federal or State law? ☐ Yes ☐ No

9. Managing/Directing Employees

If applicant is the sole owner and the sole managing/directing employee, skip this section.

Check here ☐ if deleting this managing/directing employee's association with the applicant.

Effective date of deletion? _____ (MM/DD/YYYY)

What is the total number of managing/directing employees for all location(s) listed in this application? _____ (Maximum of 20)

For each managing/directing employee, complete this section. If more than one, copy and complete this section for each.

A. Identifying Information

Name: First	Middle	Last	Jr., Sr., etc.	M.D., D.O., etc.	Title/Position

Social Security Number	Employer Identification Number (if applicable)	Medicare Identification Number (if applicable)

Date of Birth (MM/DD/YYYY)	County of Birth	State of Birth	Country of Birth

Legal Name of Business
Where This Person Manages/Directs

"Doing Business As" Name
Where This Person Manages/Directs

B. Has this Managing/Directing employee ever had a Medicare or Medicaid provider number in this or any other State?

☐ Yes   ☐ No   IF YES, supply all current and prior information requested below.

If additional space is needed, copy and complete this section.

Current Carrier Name (if applicable)	Current Fiscal Intermediary Name (if applicable)	Current Medicaid Number/State (if applicable)
Prior Carrier Name (if applicable)	Prior Fiscal Intermediary Name (if applicable)	Prior Medicaid Number/State (if applicable)

9. Managing/Directing Employees (continued)

C. Has this managing/directing employee ever managed or directed other organizations that have billed or are currently billing Medicare for services? ☐ Yes ☐ No   IF YES, how many? _____

Copy and complete the following for each organization this managing/directing employee managed or directed in the last 10 years. If this list is incomplete, check here ☐ indicating that some information for the last 10 years is missing.

Legal Business Name

Medicare Identification Number	Employer Identification Number

Current Carrier Name (if applicable)	Current Fiscal Intermediary Name (if applicable)	Current Medicaid Number/State (if applicable)
Prior Carrier Name (if applicable)	Prior Fiscal Intermediary Name (if applicable)	Prior Medicaid Number/State (if applicable)

D. Has this managing/directing employee ever had ownership interest in other organizations that have billed or are currently billing Medicare for services? ☐ Yes ☐ No   IF YES, how many? _____

Copy and complete the following for each organization this managing/directing employee managed or directed in the last 10 years. If this list is incomplete, check here ☐ indicating that some information for the last 10 years is missing.

Legal Business Name

Medicare Identification Number	Employer Identification Number

Current Carrier Name (if applicable)	Current Fiscal Intermediary Name (if applicable)	Current Medicaid Number/State (if applicable)
Prior Carrier Name (if applicable)	Prior Fiscal Intermediary Name (if applicable)	Prior Medicaid Number/State (if applicable)

E. Check if this managing/directing employee has <u>ever</u> had any of the following adverse legal actions imposed by the Medicare, Medicaid, or any other federal agency or program. For each box checked, include the date the adverse legal action was imposed. Check all that apply or the "none of these" box. Attach copy of adverse legal action notification.

1.
☐ Administrative Sanction(s) _____
☐ Program exclusion(s) _____
☐ Suspension of payment(s) _____
☐ Civil monetary penalty(s) _____
☐ Assessment(s) _____
☐ Program Debarment(s) _____

2. Health Care Related:
☐ Criminal fine(s) _____
☐ Restitution order(s) _____
☐ Pending civil judgment(s) _____
☐ Pending criminal judgment(s) _____
☐ Judgment(s) pending under the False Claims Act _____

3. ☐ None of these

4. Does this managing/directing employee have any outstanding criminal fines? ☐ Yes ☐ No   restitution orders? ☐ Yes ☐ No

10. Parent/Joint Venture Information

Check here ☐ only if this entire section does not apply to the applicant.

Check if this entity is a subsidiary company or joint venture. ☐ Subsidiary Company   ☐ Joint Venture

Complete the information below about the <u>PARENT</u> company or <u>JOINT</u> venture.

Attach a copy of parent company's or other owner's IRS Form CP 575 pertaining to this applicant.

Legal Business Name

"Doing Business As" Name	Effective Date of Affiliation (MM/DD/YYYY)

Employer Identification Number	Medicare Identification Number

Current Carrier Name (if applicable)	Current Fiscal Intermediary Name (if applicable)	Current Medicaid Number/State (if applicable)
Prior Carrier Name (if applicable)	Prior Fiscal Intermediary Name (if applicable)	Prior Medicaid Number/State (if applicable)

Business Street Address Line 1

Business Street Address Line 2

City	State	ZIP Code + 4
Telephone Number	Fax Number	E-mail Address

11. Chain Organization Information

When applicable, this section to be completed by Medicare Part A institutional provider/suppliers.

Check here ☐ only if this entire section does not apply to the applicant.

Does the applicant need to register a chain action? (see list below)   ☐ Yes   ☐ No

IF YES, check the appropriate action:
☐ Applicant in chain for first time
☐ Applicant in a different chain since last report
☐ Applicant dropped out of all chains
☐ Applicant in same chain under new chain name

Complete the following information about the chain Home Office:

Name of Home Office	Effective Date of Linkage (MM/DD/YYYY)			

Name of Home Office Administrator or CEO:	First	Middle	Last	Jr., Sr., etc.	M.D., D.O., etc.

Title of Home Office Administrator

Home Office Business Street Address Line 1

Business Street Address Line 2

City	State	ZIP Code + 4

Telephone Number	Fax Number	E-mail Address

Chain Number	Name of Home Office Intermediary

Applicant's Affiliation to Chain:
☐ Joint Venture/Partnership   ☐ Managed/Related   ☐ Leased
☐ Operated/Related   ☐ Wholly Owned   ☐ Other _____

Fiscal Year End Date of this Chain (MM/DD)	Do all the providers of the chain use the same Part A fiscal intermediary? ☐ Yes ☐ No

12. Contractor Information (Business Organizations)

A. Does the applicant contract with a business organization for any medical or diagnostic services or medical supplies for which the cost or value is $10,000 or more in a 12 month period?   ☐ Yes   ☐ No

IF YES, how many business organizations does the applicant contract with? _____

For each of these contractors, complete this section. If more than one contractor, copy and complete this section for each.

B. Will the applicant be billing and receiving payment (reassigned benefits) for medical or diagnostic services or medical supplies rendered by any other business organization, (excluding individuals), regardless of cost or value?   ☐ Yes   ☐ No

IF YES, how many business organizations reassign benefits to the applicant? _____

Each business organization (excluding individuals) that reassigns benefits to the applicant must also complete the Reassignment of Benefits Statement section. If more than one reassignee, copy and complete both sections for each reassignee.

Check here ☐ if no longer using this contractor OR here ☐ if no longer accepting reassigned benefits from this business.

Legal Business Name

Doing Business As Name	Effective Date of Relationship/Reassignment (MM/DD/YYYY)

Business Street Address Line 1

Business Street Address Line 2

City	State	ZIP Code + 4

Telephone Number	Fax Number	E-mail Address

Employer Identification Number	Medicare Identification Number (if applicable)

12. Contractor Information (Business Organizations) (continued)

C. Does this business/contractor now have or ever had a Medicare or Medicaid provider number in this or any other State?
☐ Yes ☐ No IF YES, supply all current and prior information requested below.

Current Carrier Name (if applicable)	Current Fiscal Intermediary Name (if applicable)	Current Medicaid Number/State (if applicable)
Prior Carrier Name (if applicable)	Prior Fiscal Intermediary Name (if applicable)	Prior Medicaid Number/State (if applicable)

D. Check if this business/contractor has <u>ever</u> had any of the following adverse legal actions imposed by the Medicare, Medicaid, or any other federal agency or program. For each box checked, include the date the adverse legal action was imposed. Check all that apply or the "none of these" box. Attach copy of adverse legal action notification.

1.
☐ Administrative Sanction(s) _____
☐ Program exclusion(s) _____
☐ Suspension of payment(s) _____
☐ Civil monetary penalty(s) _____
☐ Assessment(s) _____
☐ Program Debarment(s) _____

2. Health Care Related:
☐ Criminal fine(s) _____
☐ Restitution order(s) _____
☐ Pending civil judgment(s) _____
☐ Pending criminal judgment(s) _____
☐ Judgment(s) pending under the False Claims Act _____

3.
☐ None of these
_____
_____
_____

4. Does this business/contractor have any outstanding criminal fines? ☐ Yes ☐ No restitution orders? ☐ Yes ☐ No

13. Reassignment of Benefits Statement (Business Organizations and Groups Only)

Check here ☐ only if this entire section does not apply to the applicant.

Medicare law prohibits payment for services to entities other than the provider/supplier who provided the services unless the provider/supplier specifically authorizes another entity (employer, facility, health care delivery system, or agent) to bill for its services, per Federal Regulation 42 CFR 424.80. This Reassignment of Benefits Statement authorizes this applicant to receive Medicare payments on your behalf.
Your contract with the applicant must be in compliance with HCFA regulations. The Reassignment of Benefits Statement must be signed by all providers/suppliers who allow this applicant to receive payment for the provider/supplier's services.

I acknowledge that, under the terms of my contract, _____
(Legal Business Name of Applicant)
is entitled to claim or receive any fees or charges for my services.

Legal Business Name of Reassignee			Reassignee's Medicare Identification Number		
Name of Authorized Representative for the Reassignee (printed) First	Middle	Last		Jr., Sr., etc.	M.D., D.O., etc.
Signature of Authorized Representative for the Reassignee (First, Middle, Last, Jr., Sr., M.D., D.O., etc.)			Date (MM/DD/YYYY)		

14. Billing Agency/Management Service Organization Address

Check here ☐ only if this entire section does not apply to the applicant.

Check here ☐ if deleting (no longer using) this billing agency/service management organization.

Applicant MUST submit a copy of the applicant's current signed billing agreement or contract with this application.

Name of Billing Agency/Management Service Organization			Employer Identification Number	
Agency/Organization Contact Person Name: First	Middle	Last		Jr., Sr., etc.
Business Street Address Line 1				
Business Street Address Line 2				
City	State		ZIP Code + 4	
Telephone Number	Fax Number		E-mail Address	

15. Electronic Claims Submission Information

Check here ☐ only if this entire section does not apply to the applicant.

Furnish the name of a contact person in this section if the applicant would like to submit claims electronically.

Contact Person Name:	First	Middle	Last	Jr., Sr., etc.

Mailing Address Line 1

Mailing Address Line 2

City	State	ZIP Code + 4
Telephone Number	Fax Number	E-mail Address

16. Surety Bond Information

Check here ☐ only if this entire section does not apply to the applicant.

Name of Surety Bond Company

Agent's Name:	First	Middle	Last	Jr., Sr., etc.
Telephone Number			Fax Number	

Amount of Surety Bond	Effective Date of Surety Bond	Annual Renewal Date of Surety Bond
$	(MM/DD/YYYY)	(MM/DD/YYYY)

17. Contact Person

Furnish the name and telephone number of a person who can answer questions about the information furnished in this application.

Name:	First	Middle	Last	Jr., Sr., etc.
Telephone Number	Fax Number		E-mail Address	

Penalties for Falsifying Information on the Medicare Health Care Provider/Supplier Enrollment Application.

1. 18 U.S.C. § 1001 authorizes criminal penalties against an individual who in any matter within the jurisdiction of any department or agency of the United States knowingly and willfully falsifies, conceals or covers up by any trick, scheme or device a material fact, or makes any false, fictitious or fraudulent statements or representations, or makes any false writing or document knowing the same to contain any false, fictitious or fraudulent statement or entry.
Individual offenders are subject to fines of up to $250,000 and imprisonment for up to five years. Offenders that are organizations are subject to fines of up to $500,000. 18 U.S.C. § 3571. Section 3571(d) also authorizes fines of up to twice the gross gain derived by the offender if it is greater than the amount specifically authorized by the sentencing statute.

2. Section 1128B(a)(1) of the Social Security Act authorizes criminal penalties against an individual who "knowingly and willfully makes or causes to be made any false statement or representation of a material fact in any application for any benefit or payment under a program under a Federal health care program."
The offender is subject to fines of up to $25,000 and/or imprisonment for up to five years.

3. The Civil False Claims Act, 31 U.S.C. § 3729 imposes civil liability, in part, on any person who:
a.) knowingly presents, or causes to be presented, to an officer or an employee of the United States Government a false or fraudulent claim for payment or approval;
b.) knowingly makes, uses, or causes to be made or used, a false record or statement to get a false or fraudulent claim paid or approved by the Government; or
c.) conspires to defraud the Government by getting a false or fraudulent claim allowed or paid.
The Act imposes a civil penalty of $5,000 to $10,000 per violation, plus 3 times the amount of damages sustained by the Government.

4. Section 1128A(a)(1) of the Social Security Act imposes civil liability, in part, on any person (including an organization, agency or other entity) that knowingly presents or causes to be presented to an officer, employee, or agent of the United States, or of any department or agency thereof, or of any State agency. . .
a claim. . .that the Secretary determines is for a medical or other item or service that the person knows or should know:
a.) was not provided as claimed; and/or
b.) the claim is false or fraudulent.
This provision authorizes a civil monetary penalty of up to $10,000 for each item or service, an assessment of up to 3 times the amount claimed, and exclusion from participation in the Medicare program and State health care programs.

5. The government may assert common law claims such as "common law fraud," "money paid by mistake," and "unjust enrichment."
Remedies include compensatory and punitive damages, restitution and recovery of the amount of the unjust profit.

HCFA 855 (1/98)
9

18. Certification Statement

I, the undersigned, certify to the following:

1.) I have read the contents of the application and the information contained herein is true, correct, and complete. If I become aware that any information in this application is not true, correct, or complete, I agree to notify the Medicare or other federal health care program contractor of this fact immediately.

2.) I authorize the Medicare or other federal health care program contractor to verify the information contained herein. I agree to notify the Medicare or other federal health care program contractor of any changes in this form within 30 days of the effective date of the change. I understand that a change in the incorporation of my organization or my status as an individual or group biller may require a new application.

3.) I have read and understand the Penalties for Falsifying Information on the Medicare Health Care Provider/Supplier Enrollment Application, as printed in this application. I am aware that falsifying information will result in fines and/or imprisonment.

4.) I am familiar with and agree to abide by the Medicare or other federal health care program laws, regulations and program instructions that apply to my provider/supplier type. The Medicare laws, regulations and instructions are available through the Medicare Contractor. I understand that payment of a claim by Medicare or other federal health care programs is conditioned on the claim and the underlying transaction complying with such laws, regulations and program instructions (including the anti-kickback statute and the Stark law), and on a provider/supplier being in compliance with any applicable conditions of participation in any federal health care program.

5.) Neither I, as an individual practitioner-nor any owner, director, officer, or employee of the company or other organization on whose behalf I am signing this certification statement, or any contractor retained by the company or any of the aforementioned persons, currently is subject to sanction under the Medicare or Medicaid program or debarred, suspended or excluded under any other Federal agency or program, or otherwise is prohibited from providing services to Medicare or other federal health care program beneficiaries.

6.) I agree that any existing or future overpayment to me by the Medicare or other federal health care program(s) may be recouped by Medicare or the other federal health care program(s) through withholding future payments.

7.) I understand that only the Medicare or other federal health care program(s) billing number for the provider/supplier who performed the service or to whom benefits were reassigned under current Medicare or other federal health care program(s) regulations may be used when billing Medicare or other federal health care program(s) for services.

8.) I understand that any omission, misrepresentation or falsification of any information contained in this application or contained in any communication supplying information to Medicare or other federal health care program(s) to complete or clarify this application may be punishable by criminal, civil, or other administrative actions including revocation of Medicare or other federal health care program(s) billing number(s), fines, penalties, damages, and/or imprisonment under Federal law.

9.) I will not knowingly present or cause to be presented a false or fraudulent claim for payment by the Medicare or other federal health care programs, and will not submit claims with deliberate ignorance or reckless disregard of their truth or falsity.

10.) I further certify that I am the individual practitioner who is applying for the billing number, or in the case of a business organization, I am an officer, chief executive officer, or general partner of the business organization that is applying for the Medicare or other federal health care program(s) billing number.

Applicant Name (printed) First		Middle	Last	Jr., Sr., etc.	M.D., D.O., etc.
Applicant Signature (First, Middle, Last, Jr., Sr., M.D., D.O., etc.)				Date (MM/DD/YYYY)	

FOR GROUPS AND ORGANIZATIONS: (Please list all "Authorized Representatives" for this group/organization)

Check here ☐ if deleting this representative from this entity.

Authorized Representative Name (printed) First		Middle	Last	Jr., Sr., etc.	M.D., D.O., etc.
Title/Position	Social Security Number			Medicare Identification Number (if applicable)	
Authorized Representative (First, Middle, Last, Jr., Sr., M.D., D.O., etc.) Signature				Date (MM/DD/YYYY)	

Check here ☐ if deleting this representative from this entity.

Authorized Representative Name (printed) First		Middle	Last	Jr., Sr., etc.	M.D., D.O., etc.
Title/Position	Social Security Number			Medicare Identification Number (if applicable)	
Authorized Representative (First, Middle, Last, Jr., Sr., M.D., D.O., etc.) Signature				Date (MM/DD/YYYY)	

Ambulance Service Suppliers

---

1. State License Information

Is applicant licensed as a Supplier of Ambulance Services by applicant's State? ☐ Yes ☐ No
IF YES, complete this section and attach a copy of the applicant's current State license.

License Number	Issuing State	Effective Date (MM/DD/YYYY)	Expiration Date (MM/DD/YYYY)

---

2. Description of Vehicle

Copy and complete this section as needed for additional vehicles.
For each vehicle, attach copy of the vehicle registration.

1. Type (automobile, aircraft, boat, etc.)	Vehicle Identification Number

Make	Model	Year (YYYY)

Does this vehicle have the following:

first aid supplies? ☐ Yes ☐ No   other safety/life saving equipment? ☐ Yes ☐ No
oxygen equipment? ☐ Yes ☐ No   two-way telecommunications radio? ☐ Yes ☐ No
warning lights? ☐ Yes ☐ No   mobile communication? ☐ Yes ☐ No
sirens? ☐ Yes ☐ No

List other medical equipment this vehicle carries.

_____   _____
_____   _____
_____   _____
_____   _____

Does this vehicle provide:

basic life support (BLS)? ☐ Yes ☐ No   land ambulance? ☐ Yes ☐ No
advanced life support (ALS)? ☐ Yes ☐ No   air ambulance? ☐ Yes ☐ No
emergency runs? ☐ Yes ☐ No   marine ambulance? ☐ Yes ☐ No
non-emergency runs? ☐ Yes ☐ No

How many crew members accompany this vehicle on runs? _____

2. Type (automobile, aircraft, boat, etc.)	Vehicle Identification Number

Make	Model	Year (YYYY)

Does this vehicle have the following:

first aid supplies? ☐ Yes ☐ No   other safety/life saving equipment? ☐ Yes ☐ No
oxygen equipment? ☐ Yes ☐ No   two-way telecommunications radio? ☐ Yes ☐ No
warning lights? ☐ Yes ☐ No   mobile communication? ☐ Yes ☐ No
sirens? ☐ Yes ☐ No

List other medical equipment this vehicle carries.

_____   _____
_____   _____
_____   _____
_____   _____

Does this vehicle provide:

basic life support (BLS)? ☐ Yes ☐ No   land ambulance? ☐ Yes ☐ No
advanced life support (ALS)? ☐ Yes ☐ No   air ambulance? ☐ Yes ☐ No
emergency runs? ☐ Yes ☐ No   marine ambulance? ☐ Yes ☐ No
non-emergency runs? ☐ Yes ☐ No

How many crew members accompany this vehicle on runs? _____

STF MM0017F.11

3. Qualification of Crew

Copy and complete this section as needed for additional crew.

1. Name:	First	Middle	Last	Jr., Sr., etc.	M.D., D.O., etc.	Social Security Number

List training completed by this crew member (i.e., First Aid, CPR, ACLS, etc.) and attach copy(s) of training certificate(s).

2. Name:	First	Middle	Last	Jr., Sr., etc.	M.D., D.O., etc.	Social Security Number

List training completed by this crew member (i.e., First Aid, CPR, ACLS, etc.) and attach copy(s) of training certificate(s).

3. Name:	First	Middle	Last	Jr., Sr., etc.	M.D., D.O., etc.	Social Security Number

List training completed by this crew member (i.e., First Aid, CPR, ACLS, etc.) and attach copy(s) of training certificate(s).

4. Billing Method

A. Certified Basic Life Support (BLS) companies complete the following:

Contact the local Medicare contractor for information on the billing method that applies in the State where applicant will operate.

Does company bill Method 1 (an all-inclusive base rate)? ☐ Yes ☐ No

Does company bill Method 2 (base rate plus a separate charge for mileage)? ☐ Yes ☐ No

Does company bill Method 3 (base rate plus a separate charge for supplies)? ☐ Yes ☐ No

Does company bill Method 4 (separate charges for services, mileage, and supplies)? ☐ Yes ☐ No

Is company certified to perform defibrillation? (IF YES, attach certification.) ☐ Yes ☐ No

Does company provide Advanced Life Support (ALS) Services under contract with a paramedic or Emergency Medical Technician (EMT) organization or an Advanced Life Support (ALS) ambulance supplier? ☐ Yes ☐ No

IF YES, submit a copy(s) of the signed contractual agreement(s).

Does the company provide Paramedic Intercept Service? ☐ Yes ☐ No

IF YES, does the Basic Life Support Service submit Medicare claims for the paramedic service (reassign benefits)? ☐ Yes ☐ No

IF YES, complete the Reassignment of Benefits Statement section.

AIR AMBULANCE ONLY: Do you bill nautical mileage ☐ or statute mileage ☐ ?

Medical Director Name:	First	Middle	Last	Jr., Sr., etc.	M.D., D.O., etc.

Social Security Number	Medicare Identification Number (if applicable)

What geographic area does company serve?

4. Billing Method (continued)

B. Certified Advanced Life Support (ALS) companies complete the following:

Contact the local Medicare contractor for information on the billing method that applies in the State where applicant will operate.

Does company bill Method 1 (an all-inclusive base rate)?	☐ Yes	☐ No
Does company bill Method 2 (base rate plus a separate charge for mileage)?	☐ Yes	☐ No
Does company bill Method 3 (base rate plus a separate charge for supplies)?	☐ Yes	☐ No
Does company bill Method 4 (separate charges for services, mileage, and supplies)?	☐ Yes	☐ No
Does company have a contract with any municipality?	☐ Yes	☐ No
IF YES, submit copy(s) of the signed contractual agreement(s).		
Is company certified to perform defibrillation? (IF YES, attach certification.)	☐ Yes	☐ No

AIR AMBULANCE ONLY: Do you bill nautical mileage ☐ or statute mileage ☐ ?

Medical Director Name:	First	Middle	Last	Jr., Sr., etc.	M.D., D.O., etc.
Social Security Number			Medicare Identification Number (if applicable)		

What geographic area does company serve?

5. Exclusion/Sanction Information

Check here ☐ only if this entire section does not apply to the applicant.

Copy and complete this section as needed for additional crew members.

If any member of the ambulance crew has <u>ever</u> had any of the following adverse legal actions imposed by the Medicare, Medicaid, or any other federal agency or program, furnish identifying information below and check the appropriate box(es). For each box checked, include the date the adverse legal action was imposed. Attach copy of adverse legal action notification.

Name:	First	Middle	Last	Jr., Sr., etc.	M.D., D.O., etc.
Social Security Number		Employer Identification Number			

1.
   ☐ Administrative Sanction(s) _____
   ☐ Program exclusion(s) _____
   ☐ Suspension of payment(s) _____
   ☐ Civil monetary penalty(s) _____
   ☐ Assessment(s) _____
   ☐ Program Debarment(s) _____

2. Health Care Related:
   ☐ Criminal fine(s) _____
   ☐ Restitution order(s) _____
   ☐ Pending civil judgment(s) _____
   ☐ Pending criminal judgment(s) _____
   ☐ Judgment(s) pending under the False Claims Act _____

3. Does this ambulance crew member have any outstanding criminal fines? ☐ Yes ☐ No   restitution orders? ☐ Yes ☐ No

Independent Diagnostic Testing Facility (IDTFs)

This attachment must be completed for each IDTF owned and/or operated by the applicant.

1. Identification of Practice Location

A. Is this practice location a mobile unit? ☐ YES ☐ NO

IF YES, please list the vehicle(s) identification number(s) and the expiration date of the license for all mobile units and submit copies of all vehicle(s) registration(s).

Vehicle Identification Number

1 _____

2 _____

3 _____

Expiration Date of License (MM/DD/YYYY)

_____

_____

_____

B. Identify the practice location for which this attachment is being completed.
If this practice location is a mobile unit, complete the address information below with the storage location of the mobile unit.

"Doing Business As" Name of This Practice Location

Practice Location Street Address Line 1

Practice Location Street Address Line 2

City	State	ZIP Code + 4

C. Is this practice location used for any other purpose? ☐ YES ☐ NO

IF YES, please answer the following questions:

Is this practice location used for another type of business? ☐ YES ☐ NO

IF YES, what type? _____

Is this practice location used for residential purposes? ☐ YES ☐ NO

IF YES, explain reason for dual use as residence. _____

If used for any purpose other than another business or a residence, please explain the other use below.

_____

D. Are all diagnostic tests and/or services performed at the practice location? ☐ YES ☐ NO

IF NO, furnish the additional location address information where the diagnostic tests and/or services are performed. If more than one location, copy and complete this section for each.

Legal Business Name

"Doing Business As" Name

Street Address Line 1

Street Address Line 2

City	State	ZIP Code + 4

Telephone Number	Fax Number	E-mail Address

2. Identification of Supervising/Directing Physician(s)

List all supervising/directing physicians affiliated with this IDTF.
For each additional supervising/directing physician, copy and complete this section.

A. Name: First	Middle	Last	Jr., Sr., etc.	M.D., D.O., etc.

Social Security Number	Medicare Identification Number

Current Medicaid Number/State (if applicable)	Prior Medicaid Number/State (if applicable)

B. Name: First	Middle	Last	Jr., Sr., etc.	M.D., D.O., etc.

Social Security Number	Medicare Identification Number

Current Medicaid Number/State (if applicable)	Prior Medicaid Number/State (if applicable)

3. Service Performance (For each additional CPT-4 or HCPCS code, copy and complete this section.)

A. List all Current Procedural Terminology, Version 4 (CPT-4) codes or HCFA Common Procedure Coding System codes (HCPCS), equipment, and model number of equipment which this facility or its contractors intend to perform, supervise, interpret, or bill.

	CPT-4 or HCPCS Code	Equipment	Model Number
1			
2			
3			
4			
5			

Where will these services be rendered? (Check all that apply.) ☐ Physician's Office ☐ Skilled Nursing Facility ☐ Hospital
☐ Other (Explain.) _____

Will this IDTF be billing for the professional services? ☐ YES ☐ NO
IF YES, fill out the following information for each physician who will be performing the professional services (interpretations).

1. Name: First	Middle	Last	Jr., Sr., etc.	M.D., D.O., etc.

Title	Social Security Number	Medicare Identification Number

2. Name: First	Middle	Last	Jr., Sr., etc.	M.D., D.O., etc.

Title	Social Security Number	Medicare Identification Number

B. Will tests be taken by employees who are licensed or approved by the State in:

X-Ray Technology ☐ YES ☐ NO   Other ☐ YES ☐ NO
Nursing ☐ YES ☐ NO   (IF YES to "Other", explain and give qualifications below.)

IF YES to any of the above, provide the following information for each employee licensed or approved and a copy of their license or certificate approval. If additional space is needed, copy and complete this section.

1. Name: First	Middle	Last	Jr., Sr., etc.	M.D., D.O., etc.

Social Security Number	License Number	License Issue Date (MM/DD/YYYY)

2. Name: First	Middle	Last	Jr., Sr., etc.	M.D., D.O., etc.

Social Security Number	License Number	License Issue Date (MM/DD/YYYY)

4. Referral Records

Does applicant maintain records of:

the name of the attending or consulting physician who ordered the test(s)? ☐ YES ☐ NO

a copy of the physician's written order(s) for the test(s)? ☐ YES ☐ NO

the name(s) of the technician(s) who rendered the service(s)? ☐ YES ☐ NO

IF YES to any of the above, explain how the referral records are maintained (e.g., electronic, paper, by patient name, by physician name).

_____

_____

_____

5. Supervising/Directing Physician Exclusion/Sanction Information

Check if this supervising/directing physician has <u>ever</u> had any of the following adverse legal actions imposed by the Medicare, Medicaid, or any other federal agency or program. For each box checked, include the date the adverse legal action was imposed. Check all that apply or the "none of these" box. Attach copy of adverse legal action notification.

A.   ☐ Administrative Sanction(s) _____   B. Health Care Related: C. ☐ None of these

☐ Program exclusion(s) _____   ☐ Criminal fine(s) _____

☐ Suspension of payment(s) _____   ☐ Restitution order(s) _____

☐ Civil monetary penalty(s) _____   ☐ Pending civil judgment(s) _____

☐ Assessment(s) _____   ☐ Pending criminal judgment(s) _____

☐ Program Debarment(s) _____   ☐ Judgment(s) pending under the False Claims Act _____

D. Does this supervising/directing physician have any outstanding criminal fines? ☐ Yes ☐ No   restitution orders? ☐ Yes ☐ No

6. Signature of Supervising/Directing Physician(s)

<u>Each</u> supervising/directing physician must sign the following statement:
For additional supervising/directing physician signatures, copy and complete this section.

I hereby acknowledge that I have agreed to provide (IDTF Name) _____ _with general supervisory and/or directing responsibilities for tests performed by this facility. If I terminate my relationship with this IDTF, I will report the date of termination to the Medicare contractor within 30 days of termination._

1. Supervising/Directing Physician First	Middle	Last	Jr., Sr., etc.	M.D., D.O., etc.	Date
Name (printed):					(MM/DD/YYYY)
Signature of Supervising/Directing Physician	(First, Middle, Last, Jr., Sr., M.D., D.O., etc.)			Title/Position	

I hereby acknowledge that I have agreed to provide (IDTF Name) _____ _with general supervisory and/or directing responsibilities for tests performed by this facility. If I terminate my relationship with this IDTF, I will report the date of termination to the Medicare contractor within 30 days of termination._

2. Supervising/Directing Physician First	Middle	Last	Jr., Sr., etc.	M.D., D.O., etc.	Date
Name (printed):					(MM/DD/YYYY)
Signature of Supervising/Directing Physician	(First, Middle, Last, Jr., Sr., M.D., D.O., etc.)			Title/Position	

ATTACHMENT 3

Home Health Agencies (HHAs)

1. Other Related Business Interests (Control and/or Ownership)

For each owner listed in the Ownership section, each managing/directing employee listed in the Managing/Directing Employee section, as well as the home health agency (HHA) itself, complete the following information about all other businesses that each owner, managing/directing employee, or the HHA has a 5% or greater ownership and/or control interest. Indicate the relationship to the HHA.

Check here ☐ if this entire attachment does not apply to the HHA, any of its owners and/or managing/directing employees.

For each owner, managing/directing employee and/or when additional space is needed, copy and complete this attachment.

Name: First	Middle	Last	Jr., Sr., etc.	M.D., D.O., etc.

Is this individual an owner or managing/directing employee? ☐ owner ☐ managing/directing employee

A. Legal Business Name of Related Business	Type of Business
"Doing Business As" Name	Employer Identification Number

Business Street Address Line 1

Business Street Address Line 2

City	State	ZIP Code + 4
Telephone Number	Fax Number	E-mail Address

Relationship of This Business to the HHA (e.g., affiliate, contractor, supplier, etc.)	Effective Date of Ownership (MM/DD/YYYY)

B. Legal Business Name of Related Business	Type of Business
"Doing Business As" Name	Employer Identification Number

Business Street Address Line 1

Business Street Address Line 2

City	State	ZIP Code + 4
Telephone Number	Fax Number	E-mail Address

Relationship of This Business to the HHA (e.g., affiliate, contractor, supplier, etc.)	Effective Date of Ownership (MM/DD/YYYY)

C. Legal Business Name of Related Business	Type of Business
"Doing Business As" Name	Employer Identification Number

Business Street Address Line 1

Business Street Address Line 2

City	State	ZIP Code + 4
Telephone Number	Fax Number	E-mail Address

Relationship of This Business to the HHA (e.g., affiliate, contractor, supplier, etc.)	Effective Date of Ownership (MM/DD/YYYY)

OMB Approval No. 0938-0685

MEDICARE

AND OTHER FEDERAL HEALTH CARE PROGRAM

CHANGE OF INFORMATION

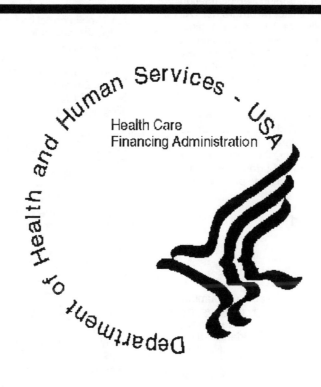

Health Care
Financing Administration

Health Care
Provider/Supplier Application

HCFA 855C (1/98)

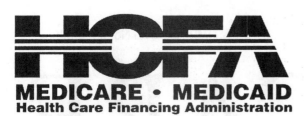

MEDICARE AND OTHER FEDERAL HEALTH CARE PROGRAMS PROVIDER/SUPPLIER FORM CHANGE OF INFORMATION INSTRUCTIONS
Change of Information Form-HCFA 855C

Upon completion, return this form and all **necessary** documentation to:

General

This form is for reporting changes in provider/supplier information for Medicare or any other federal health care programs. All changes must be requested in writing and have an original signature. Faxed or photocopied signatures will not be accepted. Changes on this form are those made most frequently and may also be reported using HCFA Form 855, 855R, or 855S, as appropriate. All changes **not** on this form **must** be reported using HCFA Forms 855, 855R, or 855S.

This form is not to be used to report a change of ownership (CHOW) as defined in 42 CFR § 489.18. A change of ownership requires the new owner to submit a completed HCFA Form 855 (General Enrollment Application). However, the current owner should complete the Potential Termination of Current Ownership section of this form to report that a potential change of ownership may occur.

Check Type of Change Being Reported

Check all changes that apply.

1. Provider/Supplier Identification

Complete provider/supplier's full name, social security number and employer identification number <u>as it is currently on file at the Medicare or other federal health care contractor</u>. The current Medicare or other federal health care program identification number must be provided (e.g. UPIN, NSC, OSCAR, PIN, NPI).

For legal business name, supply the name that the individual or entity uses in reporting to the Internal Revenue Service (IRS), as well as the individual's or entity's employer identification number (EIN) <u>as it is currently on file at the Medicare or other federal health care contractor</u>. If the EIN has changed, a new enrollment application (HCFA Form 855 or 855S) must be completed.

2. Name Change Information

If the provider/supplier is reporting a name change, complete applicable changes to the individual, organization or group name, and/or the "doing business as" name in the appropriate section. If an organization or group is requesting a name change, an IRS Form CP 575 or other official IRS correspondence must be submitted showing the new name and the tax identification number related to the new name.

3. Address/Telephone Number Change Information

Complete provider/supplier's new mailing address. This is where the provider/supplier receives notices from the Health Care Financing Administration or other federal health care programs.

Complete the "Pay To" address section if provider/supplier would like payments to go to an address other than the reported "Pay To" address currently on file. This address may be a Post Office box.

If the provider/supplier is reporting a billing agency or management service organization address change, complete identifying information for the current agency or organization and furnish the new address. If the provider/supplier is reporting a **NEW** billing agency or management service organization, do not use this form. Provider/supplier must complete the Provider/Supplier Identification and Billing Agency/Management Service Organization Address sections in the HCFA Form 855 (General Enrollment Application) and submit a copy of the new billing agreement or contract.

If provider/supplier is changing the location of the current practice, complete all information requested for the new location where provider/supplier will render services to Medicare or other federal health care program beneficiaries. If establishing a concurrent location (in addition to the current location), a new HCFA Form 855 (General Enrollment Application) must be completed for the **new** location. If deleting a current practice location, check the appropriate box.

A Post Office box or drop box is **not** acceptable as a practice location address. The phone number must be a number where patients and/or customers can reach the provider/supplier to ask questions or register complaints.

Indicate whether patient records are kept at the new practice location. If records are not kept at the new practice location, supply the physical address where the records are maintained. A Post Office or drop box address is **not** acceptable for records storage.

4. Provider/Supplier Specialty

Complete this section if provider/supplier's primary and/or secondary specialty is changing.

5. Medicare or Other Federal Health Care Program Billing Number Deactivation Information

If the provider/supplier wishes to deactivate his/her Medicare or other federal health care program billing number, identify the type of Medicare or other federal health care program billing number (e.g. UPIN, NSC, OSCAR, CHAMPUS) and provide the billing number, the effective date of deactivation for that billing number, and the reason for deactivation. Provider/suppliers may deactivate any and all Medicare or other federal health care program billing numbers as necessary by listing all applicable numbers, their types, and effective dates of deactivation as outlined above. However, applicant must notify each individual federal agency regarding the deactivation of the number(s) under that agency's control.

6. Addition/Deletion of Authorized Representative

Complete this section if provider/supplier wishes to delete a currently listed authorized representative, or the provider/supplier would like to report a new authorized representative.

An Authorized Representative is the appointed official (e.g., officer, chief executive officer, general partner, etc.) who has the authority to enroll the entity in Medicare or other federal health care programs as well as to make changes and/or updates to the applicant's status, and to commit the corporation to Medicare or other federal health care program laws and regulations.

The original signature of the new authorized representative is required to add a new authorized representative.

7. Surety Bond Information

This section to be completed by all providers/suppliers for which a surety bond is required.

Annual renewals must be reported to the Medicare or other federal health care program contractor using this Change of Information form - HCFA Form 855C.

An original copy of the surety bond must be submitted with this form. Failure to submit an original copy of the surety bond will prevent the processing of this form. In addition, the surety bond company must submit a certified copy of the agent's Power of Attorney with this form, if the bond is issued by an agent.

> Note: It is the responsibility of the provider/supplier to obtain and submit with this form a certified copy of the surety bond agent's Power of Attorney from the surety bond company, if the bond is issued by an agent.

8. Potential Termination of Current Ownership

When a business or organization is planning a change of ownership which is in accordance with the provisions for Change of Ownership (CHOW) as defined in 42 CFR § 489.18, the current owner must furnish the name of the potential new owner and the projected effective date of the potential change of ownership as soon as the possibility of such an action is known to the current owner.

> **Note:** This section is not to be completed when the existing business/organization is adding or deleting a new owner. Changes of individual owners should be reported using the appropriate sections of HCFA Form 855 (General Enrollment Application).

9. Effective Date of Change(s)

Report the date all listed changes are effective.

10. Attestation Statement

Sign and date this form attesting to the accuracy of the requested changes. If changes are being reported on an individual provider/supplier, then that individual provider/supplier must sign this form. If the changes are being reported for an organization or group practice, an authorized representative of the organization or group practice must sign this form to confirm the requested change(s).

THIS FORM SHOULD BE RETURNED TO YOUR LOCAL MEDICARE OR OTHER FEDERAL HEALTH CARE PROGRAM CONTRACTOR. SEE THE RETURN ADDRESS AT THE BEGINNING OF THESE INSTRUCTIONS.

MEDICARE/FEDERAL HEALTH CARE PROVIDER/SUPPLIER FORM
Change of Information Form

Type of Change
(Check all that apply.)

- ☐ Name
- ☐ "Pay To" Address
- ☐ E-Mail Address
- ☐ Potential Termination of Current Ownership

- ☐ Practice Location Address
- ☐ Billing Agency Address
- ☐ Authorized Representative

- ☐ Mailing Address
- ☐ Specialty
- ☐ Deactivation of Medicare Billing Number(s)
- ☐ Surety Bond Change or Renewal Information

- ☐ Telephone Number(s)
- ☐ Fax Number(s)

1. Provider/Supplier Identification   (Required)

Individual Name: First	Middle	Last		Jr., Sr., etc.	M.D., D.O., etc.

Other Name: First	Middle	Last		Jr., Sr., etc.	M.D., D.O., etc.

OR

Business Name:

Social Security Number (if applicable)	Employer Identification Number (if applicable)	Medicare Identification Number(s) (if applicable)

2. Name Change Information

A. Individuals ONLY

Prior Name: First	Middle	Last		Jr., Sr., etc.	M.D., D.O., etc.

New Name: First	Middle	Last		Jr., Sr., etc.	M.D., D.O., etc.

Social Security Number (if applicable)	Employer Identification Number (if applicable)	Medicare Identification Number(s) (if applicable)

B. Organizations or Groups ONLY

New Legal Business Name	Employer Identification Number

C. "Doing Business As" Name

Under what new name do you conduct business?

3. Address/Telephone Number Change Information

A. Mailing Address

New Mailing Address Line 1

New Mailing Address Line 2

New City	New State	New ZIP Code + 4
New Telephone Number ( )	New Fax Number ( )	New E-mail Address

B. "Pay To" Address

New Mailing Address Line 1

New Mailing Address Line 2

New City	New State	New ZIP Code + 4	New Telephone Number ( )

C. Billing Agency/Management Service Organization Address

Attach a copy of the most current signed contract with provider/supplier's billing agency or management service organization.

Name of Billing Agency/Management Service Organization				Employer Identification Number	

Agency/Organization Contact Person Name:	First	Middle	Last	Jr., Sr., etc.	Title

New Telephone Number ( )	New Fax Number ( )			New E-mail Address	

New Business Street Address Line 1

New Business Street Address Line 2

New City	New State	New ZIP Code + 4

D. Practice Location(s)   (For each additional location, copy and complete this section.)

Check whether adding or deleting the practice location identified below.   ☐ Adding   ☐ Deleting

New Street Address Line 1

New Street Address Line 2

New City	New County	New State	New ZIP Code + 4

New Telephone Number ( )	New Fax Number ( )	New E-mail Address

Are all patient records stored at this new practice location?   ☐ Yes   ☐ No   **IF NO, supply storage location below.**

Name of New Storage Facility/Location

New Street Address Line 1

New Street Address Line 2

New City	New County	New State	New ZIP Code + 4

New Telephone Number ( )	New Fax Number ( )	New E-mail Address

New Primary Specialty	New Secondary Specialty

Type (OSCAR, UPIN, PIN, etc.)	Medicare/Other Federal Health Care Program Number	Effective Date of Deactivation (MM/DD/YYYY)

Reason for deactivation request?

For each additional authorized representative, copy and complete this section.

☐ **Addition of Authorized Representative** Effective date (MM/DD/YYYY) _____	☐ **Deletion of Authorized Representative** Effective date (MM/DD/YYYY) _____

Authorized Representative Name: (printed)	First	Middle	Last	Jr., Sr., etc.	M.D., D.O., etc.

Title/Position	Social Security Number	Medicare Identification Number(s) (if applicable)	

Authorized Representative Signature (First, Middle, Last, Jr., Sr., M.D., D.O., etc.)	Date (MM/DD/YYYY)

7. Surety Bond Change or Renewal Information

An original copy of the current surety bond must be submitted with this section.

A certified copy of the surety bond agent's Power of Attorney must be submitted with this section.

Name of Surety Bond Company	Telephone Number ( )	Fax Number ( )

Agent's Name: First	Middle	Last	Jr., Sr., etc.

Amount of Surety Bond $	Effective Date (MM/DD/YYYY)
Bond for Tax Year:	Annual Renewal Date (MM/DD/YYYY)

8. Potential Termination of Current Ownership

Furnish name of potential new owner and projected effective date of change of ownership.

Individual Name of Potential New Owner: First	Middle	Last	Jr., Sr., etc.	M.D., D.O., etc.
OR				

Legal Business Name of Potential New Owner:

Projected Effective Date of Change of Ownership (MM/DD/YYYY)	Medicare Identification Number of Potential New Owner (if applicable)

9. Effective Date of Change(s)

This change/these changes are effective as of

_____ (MM/DD/YYYY)

10. Attestation Statement

I certify that I have examined the above information and that it is true, accurate and complete. I understand that any misrepresentation or concealment of material information may subject me to liability under civil and criminal laws.

Provider/Supplier Name: First (printed)	Middle	Last	Jr., Sr., etc.	M.D., D.O., etc.

Provider/Supplier Signature (First, Middle, Last, Jr., Sr., M.D., D.O., etc.)	Date (MM/DD/YYYY)

or for groups and organizations:

Authorized Representative Name: First (printed)	Middle	Last	Jr., Sr., etc.	M.D., D.O., etc.

Title/Position	Social Security Number	Medicare Identification Number (if applicable)

Authorized Representative Signature (First, Middle, Last, Jr., Sr., M.D., D.O., etc.)	Date (MM/DD/YYYY)

PLEASE
DO NOT
STAPLE
IN THIS
AREA

HEALTH INSURANCE CLAIM FORM

| | PICA | | | | | | | | | PICA | |

1. MEDICARE □ (Medicare #) **MEDICAID** □ (Medicaid #) **CHAMPUS** □ (Sponsor's SSN) **CHAMPVA** □ (VA File #) **GROUP HEALTH PLAN** □ (SSN or ID) **FECA BLK LUNG** □ (SSN) **OTHER** □ (ID)

1a. INSURED'S I.D. NUMBER (FOR PROGRAM IN ITEM 1)

2. PATIENT'S NAME (Last Name, First Name, Middle Initial)

3. PATIENT'S BIRTH DATE MM DD YY **SEX** M □ F □

4. INSURED'S NAME (Last Name, First Name, Middle Initial)

5. PATIENT'S ADDRESS (No., Street)

6. PATIENT RELATIONSHIP TO INSURED Self □ Spouse □ Child □ Other □

7. INSURED'S ADDRESS (No., Street)

CITY | STATE

8. PATIENT STATUS Single □ Married □ Other □
Employed □ Full-Time Student □ Part-Time Student □

CITY | STATE

ZIP CODE | TELEPHONE (Include Area Code)

ZIP CODE | TELEPHONE (INCLUDE AREA CODE)

9. OTHER INSURED'S NAME (Last Name, First Name, Middle Initial)

10. IS PATIENT'S CONDITION RELATED TO:

11. INSURED'S POLICY GROUP OR FECA NUMBER

a. OTHER INSURED'S POLICY OR GROUP NUMBER

a. EMPLOYMENT? (CURRENT OR PREVIOUS) □ YES □ NO

a. INSURED'S DATE OF BIRTH MM DD YY **SEX** M □ F □

b. OTHER INSURED'S DATE OF BIRTH MM DD YY **SEX** M □ F □

b. AUTO ACCIDENT? □ YES □ NO **PLACE (State)**

b. EMPLOYER'S NAME OR SCHOOL NAME

c. EMPLOYER'S NAME OR SCHOOL NAME

c. OTHER ACCIDENT? □ YES □ NO

c. INSURANCE PLAN NAME OR PROGRAM NAME

d. INSURANCE PLAN NAME OR PROGRAM NAME

10d. RESERVED FOR LOCAL USE

d. IS THERE ANOTHER HEALTH BENEFIT PLAN? □ YES □ NO *If yes,* return to and complete item 9 a - d.

READ BACK OF FORM BEFORE COMPLETING & SIGNING THIS FORM.
12. PATIENT'S OR AUTHORIZED PERSON'S SIGNATURE I authorize the release of any medical or other information necessary to process this claim. I also request payment of government benefits either to myself or to the party who accepts assignment below.

SIGNED _____ DATE _____

13. INSURED'S OR AUTHORIZED PERSON'S SIGNATURE I authorize payment of medical benefits to the undersigned physician or supplier for services described below.

SIGNED _____

14. DATE OF CURRENT: MM DD YY ◄ **ILLNESS (First symptom) OR INJURY (Accident) OR PREGNANCY (LMP)**

15. IF PATIENT HAS HAD SAME OR SIMILAR ILLNESS. GIVE FIRST DATE MM DD YY

16. DATES PATIENT UNABLE TO WORK IN CURRENT OCCUPATION MM DD YY MM DD YY
FROM _____ TO _____

17. NAME OF REFERRING PHYSICIAN OR OTHER SOURCE

17a. I.D. NUMBER OF REFERRING PHYSICIAN

18. HOSPITALIZATION DATES RELATED TO CURRENT SERVICES MM DD YY MM DD YY
FROM _____ TO _____

19. RESERVED FOR LOCAL USE

20. OUTSIDE LAB? □ YES □ NO **$ CHARGES**

21. DIAGNOSIS OR NATURE OF ILLNESS OR INJURY. (RELATE ITEMS 1, 2, 3 OR 4 TO ITEM 24E BY LINE)
1. └____
2. └____
3. └____
4. └____

22. MEDICAID RESUBMISSION CODE | **ORIGINAL REF. NO.**

23. PRIOR AUTHORIZATION NUMBER

24.	A					B	C	D		E	F	G	H	I	J	K
	DATE(S) OF SERVICE					Place of Service	Type of Service	PROCEDURES, SERVICES, OR SUPPLIES (Explain Unusual Circumstances)		DIAGNOSIS CODE	$ CHARGES	DAYS OR UNITS	EPSDT Family Plan	EMG	COB	RESERVED FOR LOCAL USE
	From MM DD YY			To MM DD YY				CPT/HCPCS	MODIFIER							
1																
2																
3																
4																
5																
6																

25. FEDERAL TAX I.D. NUMBER SSN □ EIN □

26. PATIENT'S ACCOUNT NO.

27. ACCEPT ASSIGNMENT? (For govt. claims, see back) □ YES □ NO

28. TOTAL CHARGE $

29. AMOUNT PAID $

30. BALANCE DUE $

31. SIGNATURE OF PHYSICIAN OR SUPPLIER INCLUDING DEGREES OR CREDENTIALS (I certify that the statements on the reverse apply to this bill and are made a part thereof.)

SIGNED _____ DATE _____

32. NAME AND ADDRESS OF FACILITY WHERE SERVICES WERE RENDERED (If other than home or office)

33. PHYSICIAN'S, SUPPLIER'S BILLING NAME, ADDRESS, ZIP CODE & PHONE #

PIN# | GRP#

(APPROVED BY AMA COUNCIL ON MEDICAL SERVICE 8/88) **PLEASE PRINT OR TYPE**

FORM HCFA-1500 (12-90), FORM RRB-1500, FORM OWCP-1500

STF MM0022F

2010.   PURPOSE OF HEALTH INSURANCE CLAIM FORM - HCFA-1500

The Form HCFA-1500 answers the needs of many health insurers. It is the basic form prescribed by HCFA for the Medicare program for claims from physicians and suppliers, except for ambulance services. It has also been adopted by the Office of Civilian Health and Medical Program of the Uniformed Services (OCHAMPUS) and has received the approval of the American Medical Association (AMA) Council on Medical Services.

Use these instructions for completing this form. The Form HCFA-1500 has space for physicians and suppliers to provide information on other health insurance. Use this information to determine whether the Medicare patient has other coverage which must be billed prior to Medicare payment, or whether there is a Medigap policy under which payments are made to a participating physician or supplier.

NOTE: Instructions in §§2010.1 and 2010.2 (see below) that require the reporting of 8-digit dates in all date of birth fields (items 3, 9b, and 11a), and either 6-digit or 8-digit dates in all other date fields (items 11b, 12, 14, 16, 18, 19, 24a, and 31) are effective for providers of service and suppliers as of 10/01/98.

Providers of service and suppliers have the option of entering either 6 or 8-digit dates in items 11b, 14, 16, 18, 19, or 24a. However, if a provider of service or supplier chooses to enter 8-digit dates for items 11b, 14, 16, 18, 19, or 24a, he or she must enter 8-digit dates for <u>all</u> these fields. For instance, a provider of service or supplier will <u>not</u> be permitted to enter 8-digit dates for items 11b, 14, 16, 18, 19 and a 6-digit date for item 24a. The same applies to providers of service and suppliers who choose to submit 6-digit dates too. Items 12 and 31 are exempt from this requirement.

LEGEND:	
MM	Month (e.g., December = 12)
DD	Day (e.g., Dec. 15 = 15)
YY	2 Position Year (e.g., 1998 = 98)
CCYY	4 Position Year (e.g., 1998 = 1998)
(MM | DD | YY) or (MM | DD | CCYY)	Indicates that a space must be reported between month, day, and year (e.g., 12 | 15 | 98 or 12 | 15 | 1998). This space is delineated by a dotted vertical line on Form HCFA-1500.
(MMDDYY) or (MMDDCCYY)	Indicates that no space must be reported between month, day, and year (e.g., 121598 or 12151998). The date must be reported as one continuous number.

2010.1   <u>Items 1-13 - Patient and Insured Information.</u>--

<u>Item 1.</u>   Show the type of health insurance coverage applicable to this claim by checking the appropriate box, e.g., if a Medicare claim is being filed, check the Medicare box.

<u>Item 1a.</u>   Enter the patient's Medicare Health Insurance Claim Number (HICN) whether Medicare is the primary or secondary payer.

Item 2.   Enter the patient's last name, first name, and middle initial, if any, as shown on the patient's Medicare card.

Item 3.   Enter the patient's 8-digit birth date (MM | DD | CCYY) and sex.

Item 4.   If there is insurance primary to Medicare, either through the patient's or spouse's employment or any other source, list the name of the insured here. When the insured and the patient are the same, enter the word SAME. If Medicare is primary, leave blank.

Item 5.   Enter the patient's mailing address and telephone number. On the first line enter the street address; the second line, the city and state; the third line, the ZIP code and phone number.

Item 6.   Check the appropriate box for patient's relationship to insured when item 4 is completed.

Item 7.   Enter the insured's address and telephone number. When the address is the same as the patient's, enter the word SAME. Complete this item only when items 4 and 11 are completed.

Item 8.   Check the appropriate box for the patient's marital status and whether employed or a student.

Item 9.   Enter the last name, first name, and middle initial of the enrollee in a Medigap policy if it is different from that shown in item 2. Otherwise, enter the word SAME. If no Medigap benefits are assigned, leave blank. This field may be used in the future for supplemental insurance plans.

NOTE: ONLY PARTICIPATING PHYSICIANS AND SUPPLIERS ARE TO COMPLETE ITEM 9 AND ITS SUBDIVISIONS AND ONLY WHEN THE BENEFICIARY WISHES TO ASSIGN HIS/HER BENEFITS UNDER A MEDIGAP POLICY TO THE PARTICIPATING PHYSICIAN OR SUPPLIER.

Participating physicians and suppliers must enter information required in item 9 and its subdivisions if requested by the beneficiary. Participating physicians/suppliers sign an agreement with Medicare to accept assignment of Medicare benefits for all Medicare patients. A claim for which a beneficiary elects to assign his/her benefits under a Medigap policy to a participating physician/supplier is called a mandated Medigap transfer.

Medigap.--A Medigap policy meets the statutory definition of a "Medicare supplemental policy" contained in §1882(g)(1) of Title XVIII of the Social Security Act and the definition contained in the NAIC Model Regulation which is incorporated by reference to the statute. It is a health insurance policy or other health benefit plan offered by a private entity to those persons entitled to Medicare benefits and is specifically designed to supplement Medicare benefits. It fills in some of the "gaps" in Medicare coverage by providing payment for some of the charges for which Medicare does not have responsibility due to the applicability of deductibles, coinsurance amounts, or other limitations imposed by Medicare. It does not include limited benefit coverage available to Medicare beneficiaries such as "specified disease" or "hospital indemnity" coverage. Also, it explicitly excludes a policy or plan offered by an employer to employees or former employees, as well as that offered by a labor organization to members or former members.

Do not list other supplemental coverage in item 9 and its subdivisions at the time a Medicare claim is filed. Other supplemental claims are forwarded automatically to the private insurer if the private insurer contracts with the carrier to send Medicare claim information electronically. If there is no such contract, the beneficiary must file his/her own supplemental claim.

Item 9a.   Enter the policy and/or group number of the Medigap insured preceded by **MEDIGAP, MG, or MGAP**.

NOTE: Item 9d must be completed if you enter a policy and/or group number in item 9a.

Item 9b.   Enter the Medigap insured's 8-digit birth date (MM | DD | CCYY) and sex.

Item 9c.   Leave blank if a Medigap PayerID is entered in item 9d. Otherwise, enter the claims processing address of the Medigap insurer. Use an abbreviated street address, two letter postal code, and zip code copied from the Medigap insured's Medigap identification card. For example:

   1257 Anywhere Street
   Baltimore, MD 21204

is shown as "1257 Anywhere St MD 21204."

Item 9d.   Enter the 9-digit PAYERID number of the Medigap insurer. If no PAYERID number exists, then enter the Medigap insurance program or plan name.

If you are a participating provider of service or supplier and the beneficiary wants Medicare payment data forwarded to a Medigap insurer under a mandated Medigap transfer, all of the information in items 9, 9a, 9b, and 9d must be complete and accurate. Otherwise, the Medicare carrier cannot forward the claim information to the Medigap insurer.

Items 10a thru 10c.   Check "YES" or "NO" to indicate whether employment, auto liability, or other accident involvement applies to one or more of the services described in item 24. Enter the State postal code. Any item checked "YES" indicates there may be other insurance primary to Medicare. Identify primary insurance information in item 11.

Item 10d. Use this item exclusively for Medicaid (MCD) information. If the patient is entitled to Medicaid, enter the patient's Medicaid number preceded by MCD.

Item 11. THIS ITEM MUST BE COMPLETED.   BY COMPLETING THIS ITEM, THE PHYSICIAN/SUPPLIER ACKNOWLEDGES HAVING MADE A GOOD FAITH EFFORT TO DETERMINE WHETHER MEDICARE IS THE PRIMARY OR SECONDARY PAYER.

If there is insurance primary to Medicare, enter the insured's policy or group number and proceed to items 11a - 11c.

NOTE: Enter the appropriate information in item 11c if insurance primary to Medicare is indicated in item 11.

If there is no insurance primary to Medicare, enter the word "NONE" and proceed to item 12.

If the insured reports a terminating event with regard to insurance which had been primary to Medicare (e.g., insured retired), enter the word "NONE" and proceed to item 11b.

Insurance Primary to Medicare.--Circumstances under which Medicare payment may be secondary to other insurance include:

   o   Group Health Plan Coverage:

        --   Working Aged;
        --   Disability (Large Group Health Plan); and
        --   End Stage Renal Disease;

   o   No Fault and/or Other Liability; and

o   Work-Related Illness/Injury:

> -- Workers' Compensation;
> -- Black Lung; and
> -- Veterans Benefits.

NOTE: For a paper claim to be considered for Medicare secondary payer benefits, a copy of the primary payer's explanation of benefits (EOB) notice must be forwarded along with the claim form.

<u>Item 11a</u>. Enter the insured's 8-digit birth date (MM | DD | CCYY) and sex if different from item 3.

<u>Item 11b</u>. Enter employer's name, if applicable. If there is a change in the insured's insurance status, e.g., retired, enter either a 6-digit (MM | DD | YY) or 8-digit (MM | DD | CCYY) retirement date preceded by the word "RETIRED."

<u>Item 11c</u>. Enter the 9-digit PAYERID number of the primary insurer. If no PAYERID number exists, then enter the <u>complete</u> primary payer's program or plan name. If the primary payer's EOB does not contain the claims processing address, record the primary payer's claims processing address directly on the EOB.

<u>Item 11d</u>. Leave blank. Not required by Medicare.

<u>Item 12</u>.   The patient or authorized representative must sign and enter either a 6-digit date (MM | DD | YY), 8-digit date (MM | DD | CCYY) , or an alphanumeric date (e.g., January 1, 1998) unless the signature is on file. In lieu of signing the claim, the patient may sign a statement to be retained in the provider, physician, or supplier file in accordance with §§3047.1 - 3047.3, Part 3 of MCM. If the patient is physically or mentally unable to sign, a representative specified in §3008, Part 3 of MCM may sign on the patient's behalf. In this event, the statement's signature line must indicate the patient's name followed by "by" the representative's name, address, relationship to the patient, and the reason the patient cannot sign.   The authorization is effective indefinitely unless patient or the patient's representative revokes this arrangement.

The patient's signature authorizes release of medical information necessary to process the claim. It also authorizes payment of benefits to the provider of service or supplier when the provider of service or supplier accepts assignment on the claim.

<u>Signature by Mark (X)</u>.   When an illiterate or physically handicapped enrollee signs by mark, a witness must enter his/her name and address next to the mark.

<u>Item 13</u>.   The signature in this item authorizes payment of mandated Medigap benefits to the participating physician or supplier if required Medigap information is included in item 9 and its subdivisions. The patient or his/her authorized representative signs this item, or the signature must be on file as a separate Medigap authorization. The Medigap assignment on file in the participating provider of service/supplier's office must be insurer specific. It may state that the authorization applies to all occasions of service until it is revoked.

2010.2   <u>Items 14-33 - Provider of Service or Supplier Information</u>.--

<u>Item 14</u>.   Enter either a 6-digit (MM | DD | YY) or 8-digit (MM | DD | CCYY) date of current illness, injury, or pregnancy. For chiropractic services, enter either a 6-digit (MM | DD | YY) or 8-digit (MM | DD | CCYY) date of the initiation of the course of treatment and enter either a 6-digit (MM | DD | YY) or 8-digit (MM | DD | CCYY) date in item 19.

Item 15. Leave blank. Not required by Medicare.

Item 16. If the patient is employed and is unable to work in current occupation, enter either a 6-digit (MM | DD | YY) or 8-digit (MM | DD | CCYY) date when patient is unable to work. An entry in this field may indicate employment related insurance coverage.

Item 17. Enter the name of the referring or ordering physician if the service or item was ordered or referred by a physician.

Referring physician is a physician who requests an item or service for the beneficiary for which payment may be made under the Medicare program.

Ordering physician is a physician who orders non-physician services for the patient such as diagnostic laboratory tests, clinical laboratory tests, pharmaceutical services, or durable medical equipment.

The ordering/referring requirement became effective January 1, 1992 and is required by §1833(q) of the Social Security Act. All claims for Medicare covered services and items that are the result of a physician's order or referral must include the ordering/referring physician's name and National Provider Identifier (NPI). This includes parenteral and enteral nutrition, immunosuppressive drug claims, and the following:

o   Diagnostic laboratory services;

o   Diagnostic radiology services;

o   Consultative services; and

o   Durable medical equipment.

Claims for other ordered/referred services not included in the preceding list must also show the ordering/referring physician's name and NPI. For example, a surgeon must complete items 17 and 17a when a physician refers the patient. When the ordering physician is also the performing physician (as often is the case with in-office clinical laboratory tests), the performing physician's name and assigned NPI must appear in items 17 and 17a.

All physicians who order or refer Medicare beneficiaries or services must obtain an NPI even though they may never bill Medicare directly. A physician who has not been assigned an NPI must contact the Medicare carrier.

When a physician extender or other limited licensed practitioner refers a patient for consultative service, the name and NPI of the physician supervising the limited licensed practitioner must appear in items 17 and 17a.

When a patient is referred to a physician who also orders and performs a diagnostic service, a separate claim form is required for the diagnostic service.

Enter the original ordering/referring physician's name and NPI in items 17 and 17a of the first claim form.

Enter the ordering (performing) physician's name and NPI in items 17 and 17a of the second claim form.

Surrogate NPIs.--If the ordering/referring physician has not been assigned an NPI, one of the surrogate NPIs listed below must be used in item 17a. The surrogate NPI used depends on the circumstances and is used only until the physician is assigned an NPI. Enter the physician's name in item 17 and the surrogate NPI in item 17a. All surrogate NPIs, with the exception of retired physicians (RET00000), are temporary and may be used only until an NPI is assigned. You must monitor claims with surrogate NPIs.

The term "physician" when used within the meaning of §1861(r) of the Social Security Act and used in connection with performing any function or action, refers to:

(1)   A doctor of medicine or osteopathy legally authorized to practice medicine and surgery by the State in which he/she performs such function or action;

(2)   A doctor of dental surgery or dental medicine who is legally authorized to practice dentistry by the State in which he/she performs such functions and who is acting within the scope of his/her license when performing such functions;

(3)   A doctor of podiatric medicine for purposes of subsections (k), (m), (p)(1), and (s) and §§1814(a), 1832(a)(2)(F)(ii), and 1835 of the Act, but only with respect to functions which he/she is legally authorized to perform as such by the State in which he/she performs them;

(4)   A doctor of optometry, but only with respect to the provision of items or services described in §1861(s) of the Act which he/she is legally authorized to perform as a doctor of optometry by the State in which he/she performs them; or

(5)   A chiropractor who is licensed as such by a State (or in a State which does not license chiropractors as such), and is legally authorized to perform the services of a chiropractor in the jurisdiction in which he/she performs such services, and who meets uniform minimum standards specified by the Secretary, but only for purposes of §§1861(s)(1) and 1861(s)(2)(A) of the Act, and only with respect to treatment by means of manual manipulation of the spine (to correct a subluxation demonstrated by X-ray to exist). For the purposes of §1862(a)(4) of the Act and subject to the limitations and conditions provided above, chiropractor includes a doctor of one of the arts specified in the statute and legally authorized to practice such art in the country in which the inpatient hospital services (referred to in §1862(a)(4) of the Act) are furnished.

Item 17a. Enter the HCFA assigned NPI of the referring/ordering physician listed in item 17. Enter only the 7-digit base number and the 1-digit check digit.

When a claim involves multiple referring and/or ordering physicians, a separate HCFA-1500 must be used for each ordering/referring physician.

Use the following surrogate NPIs for physicians who have not been assigned individual NPIs. Claims received with surrogate numbers will be tracked and possibly audited.

o   Residents who are issued an NPI in conjunction with activities outside of their residency status must use that NPI. For interns and residents without NPIs, use the eight (8) character surrogate NPI RES00000;

o   Retired physicians who were not issued an NPI may use the surrogate RET00000;

o   Physicians serving in the Department of Veterans Affairs or the U.S. Armed Services may use VAD00000;

o   Physicians serving in the Public Health or Indian Health Services may use PHS00000;

o   The law extends coverage and direct payment in non-Metropolitan Statistical Areas to practitioners who are State licensed to order medical services or refer patients to Medicare providers without the approval or collaboration of a supervising physician. Use the surrogate NPI "NPP00000" on claims involving services ordered/referred by nurse practitioners, clinical nurse specialists, or any non-physician practitioner who is State licensed to order clinical diagnostic tests; and

o   When the ordering/referring physician has not been assigned an NPI and does not meet the criteria for using one of the surrogate NPIs, the biller may use the surrogate NPI "OTH00000" until an individual NPI is assigned.

Item 18.   Enter either a 6-digit (MM | DD | YY) or 8-digit (MM | DD | CCYY) date when a medical service is furnished as a result of, or subsequent to, a related hospitalization.

Item 19.   Enter either a 6-digit (MM | DD | YY) or 8-digit (MM | DD | CCYY) date patient was last seen and the NPI of his/her attending physician when an independent physical or occupational therapist or physician providing routine foot care submits claims. For physical and occupational therapists,   entering this information certifies that the required physician certification (or recertification) is being kept on file (See §2206.1, Part 3 of MCM).

Enter either a 6-digit (MM | DD | YY) or 8-digit (MM | DD | CCYY) X-ray date for chiropractor services. By entering an X-ray date, and the initiation date for course of chiropractic treatment in item 14, you are certifying that all the relevant information requirements (including level of subluxation) of the §2251, Part 3 of MCM and §4118, Part 3 of MCM are on file along with the appropriate X-ray and all are available for carrier review.

Enter the drug's name and dosage when submitting a claim for Not Otherwise Classified (NOC) drugs.

Enter a concise description of an "unlisted procedure code" or a NOC code if one can be given within the confines of this box. Otherwise an attachment must be submitted with the claim.

Enter all applicable modifiers when modifier -99 (multiple modifiers) is entered in item 24d. If modifier -99 is entered on multiple line items of a single claim form, all applicable modifiers for each line item containing a   -99 modifier should be listed as follows: 1=(mod), where the number 1 represents the line item and "mod" represents all modifiers applicable to the referenced line item.

Enter the statement "Homebound" when an independent laboratory renders an EKG tracing or obtains a specimen from a homebound or institutionalized patient. (See §2051.1, Part 3 of MCM and §2070.1, Part 3 of MCM respectively, for the definition of "homebound" and a more complete definition of a medically necessary laboratory service to a homebound or an institutional patient.) Enter the statement, "Patient refuses to assign benefits" when the beneficiary absolutely refuses to assign benefits to a participating provider. In this case, no payment may be made on the claim.

Enter the statement, "Testing for hearing aid" when billing services involving the testing of a hearing aid(s) is used to obtain intentional denials when other payers are involved.

When dental examinations are billed, enter the specific surgery for which the exam is being performed.

Enter the specific name and dosage amount when low osmolar contrast material is billed, but only if HCPCS codes do not cover them.

Enter either a 6-digit (MM | DD | YY) or 8-digit (MM | DD | CCYY) assumed and/or relinquished date for a global surgery claim when providers share post-operative care.

Enter the statement, "Attending physician, not hospice employee" when a physician renders services to a hospice patient but the hospice providing the patient's care (in which the patient resides) does not employ the attending physician.

Enter demonstration ID number "30" for all national emphysema treatment trial claims.

Item 20. Complete this item when billing for diagnostic tests subject to purchase price limitations. Enter the purchase price under charges if the "yes" block is checked. A "yes" check indicates that an entity other than the entity billing for the service performed the diagnostic test. A "no" check indicates that "no purchased tests are included on the claim." When "yes" is annotated, item 32 must be completed. When billing for multiple purchased diagnostic tests, each test must be submitted on a separate claim form.

Item 21. Enter the patient's diagnosis/condition. All physician specialties must use an ICD-9-CM code number and code to the highest level of specificity. Enter up to 4 codes in priority order (primary, secondary condition). An independent laboratory must enter a diagnosis only for limited coverage procedures.

All narrative diagnoses for non-physician specialties must be submitted on an attachment.

Item 22. Leave blank. Not required by Medicare.

Item 23. Enter the Professional Review Organization (PRO) prior authorization number for those procedures requiring PRO prior approval.

Enter the Investigational Device Exemption (IDE) number when an investigational device is used in an FDA-approved clinical trial.

For physicians performing care plan oversight services, enter the 6-digit Medicare provider number of the home health agency (HHA) or hospice when CPT code 99375 or 99376 or HCPCS code G0064, G0065, or G0066 is billed.

Enter the 10-digit Clinical Laboratory Improvement Act (CLIA) certification number for laboratory services billed by an entity performing CLIA covered procedures.

Item 24a. Enter either a 6-digit (MM | DD | YY) or 8-digit (MMDDCCYY) date for each procedure, service, or supply. When "from" and "to" dates are shown for a series of identical services, enter the number of days or units in column G.

Item 24b. Enter the appropriate place of service code(s) from the list provided in §2010.3. Identify the location, using a place of service code, for each item used or service performed.

NOTE: When a service is rendered to a hospital inpatient, use the "inpatient hospital" code.

Item 24c. Medicare providers are not required to complete this item.

Item 24d. Enter the procedures, services, or supplies using the HCFA Common Procedure Coding System (HCPCS). When applicable, show HCPCS modifiers with the HCPCS code.

Enter the specific procedure code without a narrative description. However, when reporting an "unlisted procedure code" or a NOC code, include a narrative description in item 19 if a coherent description can be given within the confines of that box. Otherwise, an attachment must be submitted with the claim.

Item 24e. Enter the diagnosis code reference number as shown in item 21 to relate the date of service and the procedures performed to the primary diagnosis. Enter only one reference number per line item. When multiple services are performed, enter the primary reference number for each service; either a 1, or a 2, or a 3, or a 4.

If a situation arises where two or more diagnoses are required for a procedure code (e.g., pap smears), you must reference only one of the diagnoses in item 21.

Item 24f. Enter the charge for each listed service.

Item 24g. Enter the number of days or units. This field is most commonly used for multiple visits, units of supplies, anesthesia minutes, or oxygen volume. If only one service is performed, the numeral 1 must be entered.

Some services require that the actual number or quantity billed be clearly indicated on the claim form (e.g., multiple ostomy or urinary supplies, medication dosages, or allergy testing procedures). When multiple services are provided, enter the actual number provided.

For anesthesia, show the elapsed time (minutes) in item 24g. Convert hours into minutes and enter the total minutes required for this procedure.

Suppliers must furnish the units of oxygen contents except for concentrators and initial rental claims for gas and liquid oxygen systems. Rounding of oxygen contents is as follows:

   o   For stationary gas system rentals, suppliers must indicate oxygen contents in unit multiples of 50 cubic feet in item 24g, rounded to the nearest increment of 50. For example, if 73 cubic feet of oxygen were delivered during the rental month, the unit entry "01" indicating the nearest 50 cubic foot increment is entered in item 24g.

   o   For stationary liquid systems, units of contents must be specified in multiples of 10 pounds of liquid contents delivered, rounded to the nearest 10 pound increment. For example, if 63 pounds of liquid oxygen were delivered during the applicable rental month billed, the unit entry "06" is entered in item 24g.

   o   For units of portable contents only (i.e., no stationary gas or liquid system used), round to the nearest five feet or one liquid pound, respectively.

Item 24h. Leave blank. Not required by Medicare.

Item 24i. Leave blank. Not required by Medicare.

Items 24j and 24k. Enter the NPI of the performing provider of service/supplier if they are a member of a group practice.

NOTE: Enter the first 2-digits of the NPI in item 24j. Enter the remaining 6- digits of the NPI in item 24k, including the 2-digit location identifier.

When several different providers of service or suppliers within a group are billing on the same Form HCFA-1500, show the individual NPI in the corresponding line item.

Item 25. Enter your provider of service or supplier Federal Tax I.D. (Employer Identification Number) or Social Security Number. The participating provider of service or supplier Federal Tax I.D. number is required for a mandated Medigap transfer.

Item 26. Enter the patient's account number assigned by the provider of service's or supplier's accounting system. This field is optional to assist you in patient identification. As a service, any account numbers entered here will be returned to you.

Item 27. Check the appropriate block to indicate whether the provider of service or supplier accepts assignment of Medicare benefits. If MEDIGAP is indicated in block 9 and MEDIGAP payment authorization is given in item 13, the provider of service or supplier must also be a Medicare participating provider of service or supplier and must accept assignment of Medicare benefits for all covered charges for all patients.

The following providers of service/suppliers and claims can only be paid on an assignment basis:

o   Clinical diagnostic laboratory services;

o   Physician services to individuals dually entitled to Medicare and Medicaid;

o   Participating physician/supplier services,

o   Services of physician assistants, nurse practitioners, clinical nurse specialists, nurse midwives, certified registered nurse anesthetists, clinical psychologists, and clinical social workers,

o   Ambulatory surgical center services for covered ASC procedures; and

o   Home dialysis supplies and equipment paid under Method II.

Item 28. Enter total charges for the services (i.e., total of all charges in item 24f).

Item 29. Enter the total amount the patient paid on the covered services only.

Item 30. Leave blank. Not required by Medicare.

Item 31. Enter the signature of provider of service or supplier, or his/her representative, and either the 6-digit date (MM | DD | YY), 8-digit date (MM | DD | CCYY), or alphanumeric date (e.g., January 1, 1998) the form was signed.

Item 32. Enter the name and address of the facility if the services were furnished in a hospital, clinic, laboratory, or facility other than the patient's home or physician's office. When the name and address of the facility where the services were furnished is the same as the billers name and address shown in item 33, enter the word "SAME." Providers of service (namely physicians) must identify the supplier's name, address, and NPI when billing for purchased diagnostic tests. When more than one supplier is used, a separate HCFA-1500 should be used to bill for each supplier.

This item is completed whether the supplier personnel performs the work at the physician's office or at another location.

If a QB or QU modifier is billed, indicating the service was rendered in a Health Professional Shortage Area (HPSA), the physical location where the service was rendered must be entered if other than home. However, if the address shown in item 33 is in a HPSA and is the same as where the services were rendered, enter the word "SAME."

If the supplier is a certified mammography screening center, enter the 6-digit FDA approved certification number.

Complete this item for all laboratory work performed outside a physician's office. If an independent laboratory is billing, enter the place where the test was performed and the NPI, including the 2-digit location identifier.

Item 33. Enter the provider of service/supplier's billing name, address, zip code, and telephone number.

Enter the NPI, including the 2-digit location identifier, for the performing provider of service/supplier who is not a member of a group practice.

Enter the group NPI, including the 2-digit location identifier, for the performing provider of service/supplier who is a member of a group practice.

OMB Approval No. 0938-0685

MEDICARE
AND OTHER FEDERAL HEALTH CARE PROGRAM
INDIVIDUAL REASSIGNMENT OF BENEFITS

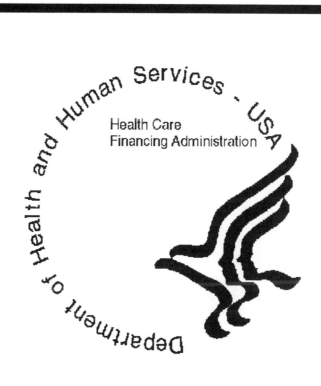

Department of Health and Human Services - USA

Health Care
Financing Administration

Health Care
Provider/Supplier Application

HCFA 855R (1/98)

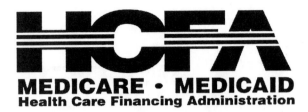

MEDICARE AND OTHER FEDERAL HEALTH CARE PROGRAMS PROVIDER/SUPPLIER ENROLLMENT APPLICATION INSTRUCTIONS
Individual Reassignment of Benefits Application
HCFA 855R

Upon completion, return this application and all necessary documentation to:

Definitions

Authorized Representative: The appointed official (e.g., officer, chief executive officer, general partner, etc.) who has the authority to enroll the entity in Medicare or other federal health care programs as well as to make changes and/or updates to the applicant's status, and to commit the corporation to Medicare or other federal health care program laws and regulations.

The Authorized Representative may be contacted to answer questions regarding the information furnished in this application.

General

This application is to be completed for any <u>individual</u> who will reassign their benefits to an eligible entity.

THIS REASSIGNMENT OF BENEFITS APPLICATION MUST BE COMPLETED FOR THE FOLLOWING SITUATIONS:

Initial Enrollment: A newly enrolling entity will complete this application for each individual who will be reassigning Medicare or other federal health care program benefits to the enrolling entity.

> **NOTE:** All entities and individuals must be currently enrolled or concurrently enrolling in the Medicare or other federal health care program in which they want to reassign their benefits.

Adding a Reassignment: An individual practitioner is currently enrolled in Medicare or another federal health care program(s) and will reassign benefits to an entity that is currently in the Medicare or the same other federal health care program(s).

Deleting a Reassignment: An individual that has been reassigning benefits to an entity is terminating that reassignment. No reassigned claims will be paid to the entity for dates of service after the effective date of deletion.

Changing Status of an Individual: An individual reporting a change in the type of income tax withholding or the practice location(s) with which he or she is associated.

Changes of Ownership (CHOW): This application is to be completed by all individual contractors, physicians, and other non-physician practitioners who will be reassigning their Medicare or other federal health care benefits to a new or a prospective new owner due to the occurrence or potential occurrence of a CHOW.

Change of Ownership (CHOW): This term applies to certain limited circumstances as defined in 42 CFR § 489.18 as described below.

A new or prospective new owner must complete this application to report new or prospective new ownership. In addition, the applicant must also submit an Individual Reassignment of Benefits Application (HCFA Form 855R) identifying all individuals who will reassign their benefits to the applicant.

A change of ownership is defined as:

- In the case of a <u>partnership</u>, the removal, addition, or substitution of a partner, unless the partners expressly agree otherwise, as permitted by applicable State law;

- In the case of an <u>unincorporated sole proprietorship</u>, transfer of title and property to another party;

- In the case of a <u>corporation</u>, the merger of the provider corporation into another corporation, or the consolidation of two or more corporations, resulting in the creation of a new corporation (transfer of corporate stock or the merger of another corporation into the provider corporation does not constitute a change of ownership); and

- In the case of <u>leasing</u>, the lease of all or part of a provider/supplier facility constitutes a change of ownership of the leased portion.

Entity: A business organization (e.g., group practice, hospital, clinic, health care delivery system) that is eligible to receive reassigned benefits as permitted under 42 CFR 424.80.

Individual: A physician or other individual practitioner who is eligible to receive Medicare or other federal health program benefits and is permitted to reassign his or her benefits to an eligible entity.

Definitions(continued)

Medicare Identification Number: This number uniquely identifies individuals and entities as Medicare providers/suppliers and is the number used on claim forms. The Medicare identification number is also known as Medicare Provider Number and Provider Identification Number (PIN). Examples of Medicare Identification Numbers are the UPIN, OSCAR number and NSC number.

National Provider Identifier (NPI): This number is assigned using the National Provider System to identify health care provider/suppliers. In the future, it will replace the Medicare Identification Number.

Reassignee: An individual or organization that allows another organization to bill Medicare or other federal health care programs on their behalf for services rendered.

APPLICATION COMPLETION INSTRUCTIONS

Check the box indicating the reason this application is being completed.

1. Entity Identification

Complete information identifying the entity to whom Medicare or other federal health care program benefits are being reassigned.

The legal business name of the entity must be the same name the entity uses in reporting to the Internal Revenue Service.

2. Individual Identification

Complete this section for each individual who is reassigning or terminating reassignment of his or her Medicare or other federal health care program benefits to the entity shown in the Entity Identification section. Indicate the type of action being reported.

> **Note:** This form may be used to add or delete an individual who is reassigning or has previously reassigned his or her benefits to the entity.

3. Practice Location(s)

Complete all information requested for each location where the individual identified in the Individual Identification section (above) will render services to Medicare or other federal health care program beneficiaries on behalf of the entity identified in the Entity Identification section. The entity must have enrolled, or be in the process of enrolling, all of these practice locations using the HCFA Form 855 (General Enrollment Application).

4. Billing Agency/Management Service Organization Address

A Billing Agency is a company contracted by the applicant to furnish all claims processing functions for the applicant's practice.

A Management Service Organization is a company contracted by the applicant to furnish some or all administrative, clerical and claims processing functions of the applicant's practice.

Complete this section if the entity shown in the Entity Identification section currently uses a billing agency and/or management service organization to submit bills.

5. Reassignment of Benefits Statement

This Reassignment of Benefits Statement must be completed when an individual practitioner will be reassigning his or her benefits to an eligible entity (employer, facility, health care delivery system, or agent).

In general, Medicare and other federal health care programs only make payments to the beneficiary or the individual or entity that directly provides the service. However, an individual may reassign benefits to an eligible entity as defined in 42 CFR 424.80.

The Legal Business Name of the entity must be the same as the Legal Business Name of the entity identified in Section 1 of this application.

The individual reassigning his or her benefits must sign this statement. Failure to complete and sign the Reassignment of Benefits Statement will cause a delay in processing the application and limit the Health Care Financing Administration's or other federal health care program's ability to make payment.

> **Note:** For further information on Federal requirements on reassignment of benefits, the reassignee should contact his or her Medicare or other federal health care program contractor before signing this application.

6. Contact Person

Provide the full name and telephone number of an individual who can be reached to answer questions regarding the information furnished in this application.

7. Attestation Statement

The Authorized Representative of the entity that will receive payments must sign and date this application, attesting to the accuracy of the information provided and certifying that the entity applying to receive payments is eligible to receive reassigned benefits.

SEE PAGE ONE OF THESE INSTRUCTIONS FOR THE ADDRESS TO RETURN THIS COMPLETED APPLICATION.

According to the Paperwork Reduction Act of 1995, no persons are required to respond to a collection of information unless it displays a valid OMB control number. The valid OMB control number for this information collection is 0938-0685. The time required to complete this information collection is estimated to average 30 minutes per response, including the time to review instructions, search existing data resources, gather the data needed, and complete and review the information collection. If you have any comments concerning the accuracy of the time estimate(s) or suggestions for improving this form, please write to: HCFA, P.O. Box 26684, Baltimore, Maryland 21207 and to the Office of Information and Regulatory Affairs, Office of Management and Budget, Washington, D.C. 20503.

MEDICARE/FEDERAL HEALTH CARE PROVIDER/SUPPLIER ENROLLMENT APPLICATION
Individual Reassignment of Benefits Application

THIS APPLICATION IS TO BE COMPLETED FOR ANY INDIVIDUAL WHO WILL REASSIGN HIS OR HER BENEFITS TO AN ELIGIBLE ENTITY.

Check box indicating the reason this application is being completed.
(Note: definitions of the following terms are found in the instructions.)

☐ Initial Enrollment   ☐ Adding a Reassignment
☐ Deleting a Reassignment   ☐ Changing Status of an Individual
☐ Changes of Ownership (CHOW)

1. Entity Identification

Legal Business Name

"Doing Business As" Name

Entity Employer Identification Number	Entity Medicare Identification Number

2. Individual Identification

Adding or Listing Individual	☐	Date Individual Reassigned Benefits (required) (MM/DD/YYYY)
Deleting Individual	☐	Date Individual Terminated Reassignment (if applicable) (MM/DD/YYYY)

Name: First	Middle	Last	Jr., Sr., etc.	M.D., D.O., etc.

Social Security Number	Medicare Identification Number	Date of Birth (MM/DD/YYYY)

Individual Primary Speciality	Individual Secondary Speciality (optional)

What income reporting form does this individual receive from the entity or the Internal Revenue Service at the end of the calendar year?
☐ W-2   ☐ 1099   ☐ 1065-K1   ☐ Other _____

3. Practice Location(s)

At how many locations does this individual render services for the entity identified above? _____
List all locations where this individual will render services for this entity.

If additional space is needed, copy page, complete this section and attach to application.

Legal Business Name For This Location

"Doing Business As" Name For This Location

Business Street Address Line 1

Business Street Address Line 2

City	County	State	ZIP Code + 4

4. Billing Agency/Management Service Organization Address

Check here ☐ only if this entire section does not apply to the applicant.

Complete this section if the <u>entity</u> is using a billing agency or management service organization.

Billing Agency/Management Service Organization Name				Employer Identification Number
Agency/Organization Contact Person <u>Name</u>: First	Middle	Last		Jr., Sr., etc.
Business Street Address Line 1				
Business Street Address Line 2				
City	State		ZIP Code + 4	
Telephone Number ( )	Fax Number ( )		E-mail Address	

5. Reassignment of Benefits Statement

Medicare law prohibits payment for services to entities other than the practitioner who provided the services unless the practitioner specifically authorizes another entity (employer, facility, health care delivery system, or agent) to receive payment for his or her services, per Federal Regulation 42 CFR 424.80. By signing this Reassignment of Benefits Statement, you are authorizing the entity identified in Section 1 to receive Medicare payments on your behalf.

Your employment or contract with this entity must be in compliance with HCFA regulations. The Reassignment of Benefits Statement must be signed by all providers, suppliers, and individuals who allow an entity (employer, facility, health care delivery system, or agent) to receive payment for your services.

I acknowledge that, under the terms of my employment or contract, _____

(Legal Business Name of Entity)

is entitled to claim or receive any fees or charges for my services.

Reassignee Name (printed) First	Middle	Last		Jr., Sr., etc.	M.D., D.O., etc.
Reassignee Signature (First, Middle, Last, Jr., Sr., M.D., D.O., etc.)			Date (MM/DD/YYYY)		

6. Contact Person

Please supply the name and telephone number of a person who can answer questions about the information furnished in this application.

<u>Name</u> First	Middle	Last		Jr., Sr., etc.	Telephone Number ( )

7. Attestation Statement

I certify that I have examined the above information and that it is true, accurate and complete. I understand that any misrepresentation or concealment of material information may subject me to liability under civil and criminal laws. I certify that the entity applying to receive payments is eligible to receive reassigned benefits.

Authorized Representative Name: (printed) First	Middle	Last		Jr., Sr., etc.	M.D., D.O., etc.
Authorized Representative Title/Position	Social Security Number		Medicare Identification Number (if applicable)		
Authorized Representative Signature (First, Middle, Last, Jr., Sr., M.D., D.O., etc.)			Date (MM/DD/YYYY)		

Appendix C

Medicare Manual Memorandum and Transmittals

1. Program Memorandum B-00-06, Matrix to Complete Provider/Supplier Enrollment Application (HCFA-855)

2. Program Memorandum B-99-16, Discontinuing the Use of Modifiers for Processing of Claims for Nurse Practitioners (NPs), Physician Assistants (PAs), and Clinical Nurse Specialists (CNSs)

3. Program Memorandum B-98-47, Discontinuing the Surrogate Unique Physician Identification Number (UPIN) NPP000 for Nurse Practitioners (NPs), Clinical Nurse Specialists (CNSs), and Physician Assistants (PAs)

4. Program Memorandum B-00-2, Payment for Teleconsultations in Rural Health Professional Shortage Areas [January 1, 2000]

5. HCFA Program Manual Transmittals

Appendix C.1

Program Memorandum B-00-6
Matrix to Complete Provider/Supplier Enrollment Application (HCFA-855)

Document No. B-00-06 — Matrix to Complete Provider/Supplier Enrollment Application (HCFA-855)

PROGRAM MEMORANDUM
CARRIERS

Department of Health and Human Services
Health Care Financing Administration
Transmittal No. B-00-06
Date: FEBRUARY 2000

This Program Memorandum re-issues Program Memorandum B-99-6, Change Request 777 dated March 1999. The only change is the discard date; all other material remains the same.

CHANGE REQUEST #777

SUBJECT: Matrix to Complete Provider/Supplier Enrollment Application (HCFA-855)

In response to questions raised at the 1998 Provider Enrollment Conference in September, we have designed the attached matrix to help you identify those fields that an applicant must complete to enroll in the Medicare program as a provider/supplier.

For those columns marked with an "X" ("if applicable"), the applicant would complete the data fields if applicable. For those columns marked with an "M" ("mandatory"), the applicant must complete the section. If an applicant does not complete a section on the application where the matrix is marked "M", contact the applicant to complete the field. The decision on how to contact the applicant, in writing or by telephone, is at your discretion. (See Medicare Carrier Manual Part 4 §1030.2.) All documentation, attachments, licensure information and signatures must be submitted as required for that supplier's specialty.

If an applicant completes a section that is not required, it is not necessary to return the application. For new individuals who are joining a group, and neither the group nor the individual were enrolled prior to Form HCFA-855, both the individual and group must complete Form HCFA-855. Form HCFA-855R is to be completed by the additional individual only. The entire group does not complete Form HCFA-855R.

NOTE: The matrix does not completely match the instructions in Form HCFA-855.

As a result of issues raised at the September conference, we are no longer requiring the following applicant types to complete the corresponding data fields:

■ individual—sections 8, 12, and 13.

■ sole proprietor—sections 8, 12, and 13.

■ organization—sections 13 and 16.

■ group—sections 1b, 12, and 13.

Inform the applicant of these changes. Attachment 2 provides you with stock language informing the applicant of the change in the application instructions.

We are making corresponding changes to MCM § 1030.1.

2 Attachments

These instructions should be implemented within your current operating budget.

This Program Memorandum may be discarded after February 1, 2001.

Contractors should contact the appropriate Regional Office with any questions. Regional Office staff may direct questions to Patti Snyder on (410) 786-5991 and Allen Gillespie on (410) 786-5996.

HCFA Pub. 60B Attachment 2

STOCK LANGUAGE

Dear Applicant:

The following information is to guide you in completing certain sections of Form HCFA-855 application for your provider/supplier type, and in some cases supersedes the "Application Completion Instructions" on page III of the application. Because of budgetary constraints we cannot change the application instructions at this time.

We are no longer requiring the following applicant types to complete the corresponding data fields:

- individual—sections 8, 12, and 13
- sole proprietor—sections 8, 12, and 13
- organization—sections 13 and 16
- group—sections 1b, 12, and 13

If an entire section is not applicable, check the box at the beginning of the section indicating the entire section is not applicable. For further instructions on how to complete the application, see Page III in the application.

All applicants must check the appropriate box next to the following:

"Type of Business"

"Applicant Enrolling As" Type

"Federal Health Program"

"Application For"

"Submit Billings"

"Enrolled in Other" Individual complete sections 1A, 1D, 2, 3, 4 (if applicable), 5, 6, 7, 9, 14, 15 (if applicable), 17, and 18.

Sole Proprietor complete sections 1A, 1B, 1D, 2, 3, 4 (if applicable), 5, 6, 7, 9, 14, 15 (if applicable), 17, and 18.

Organization complete sections 1B, 1D, 2 (if State requires license), 5, 6, 7, 8, 9, 10 (if applicable), 11 (if applicable), 12, 14, 15 (if applicable), 17, and 18.

Group complete sections 1C, 1D, 2 (if State requires license), 5, 6, 7, 8, 9, 10 (if applicable), 11 (if applicable), 14, 15, (if applicable), 17, and 18. All group members/partners must complete Form HCFA Form 855R.

Partnership complete sections 1C, 1D, 2 (if required), 5, 6, 7, 8, 9, 10 (if applicable), 11 (if applicable), 14, 15 (if applicable), 17, and 18 of the general application. For partners who reassign their benefits, they must complete Form HCFA-855R.

Mass Immunization/Roster Biller complete Sections 1b, 1d, 2 (if required), 5, 6, 7, 8, 9, 14, 15 (if applicable), 17, and 18.

Appendix C.2

Program Memorandum, B-99-16
Discontinuing the Use of Modifiers for Processing of Claims for Nurse Practitioners (NPs), Physician Assistants (PAs), and Clinical Nurse Specialists (CNSs)

Document No. B-99-16 — Discontinuing the Use of Modifiers for Processing of Claims for Nurse Practitioners (NPs), Physician Assistants (PAs), and Clinical Nurse Specialists (CNSs)

PROGRAM MEMORANDUM
CARRIERS

Department of Health and Human Services
Health Care Financing Administration
Transmittal No. B-99-16
Date: APRIL 1999

CHANGE REQUEST 437

SUBJECT: Discontinuing the Use of Modifiers for Processing of Claims for Nurse Practitioners (NPs), Physician Assistants (PAs), and Clinical Nurse Specialists (CNSs)

Background

HCFA released transmittal number B-98-50, instructing carriers to continue to require providers to report modifiers for NP, PA and CNS claims even though they were discontinued on the 1999 HCPCS database effective December 31, 1998.

Delays in changes to our Common Working File system served as the basis for requiring providers to continue to report these modifiers. Changes to the CWF system will be completed prior to April 1, 1999.

Purpose

Effective April 1, 1999, claims for NPs, PAs and CNSs rendering physician type services in certain settings will not require a modifier. Claims submitted for NP, CNS and PA services must be reported under the Practitioners Provider Identification Number (PIN). Payment for NP, CNS, and PA claims will be based on the PIN.

NOTE: A modifier will continue to be used when billing for services provided by these nonphysician practitioners when performing as assistants-at-surgery.

Effective April 1, 1999, use the assigned PIN to process claims for NPs, CNSs, and PAs rendering physician services and no longer rely upon the use of modifiers, except for assistant-at-surgery services. Except for NP, PA & CNS services furnished to patients in RHCs and FQHCs, there are no longer any restrictions on the settings in which we will pay for these services. NPs, CNSs and the employer of the PA must use the PIN in the following settings: Hospitals, Clinics, Skilled Nursing Facilities (SNFs), Home Health Agencies (HHAs),

Comprehensive Outpatient Rehabilitation Facilities (CORFs), Ambulatory Surgical Centers (ASCs), Community Mental Health Centers (CMHCs), and Hospice programs. Also, the discussion of "team visits" as stated in Medicare Carriers Manual § 4113, is no longer applicable to services furnished by NPs, PAs, and CNSs in the Skilled Nursing Facility and Nursing Facility setting. HCFA will continue to use modifiers for payment of assistant-at-surgery services.

The following modifiers will no longer be reported effective after April 1, 1999:

- AK—Nurse Practitioner, rural, team member;

- AL—Nurse Practitioner, non-rural, team member;

HCFA Pub. 60B

- AN—Physician Assistant services for other than assistant-at-surgery, non-team member;

- AU—Physician Assistant for other than assistant-at-surgery, team member;

- AV—Nurse Practitioner, rural non-team member;

- AW—Clinical Nurse Specialist, non-team member; and

- AY—Clinical Nurse Specialist, team member.

Effective April 1, 1999, providers will not be required to submit these modifiers. In fact, the discontinuance of the use of these modifiers coincides with the grace period for their deletions on the 1999 HCPCS database.

In order to recognize assistant-at-surgery services provided by a NP and CNS, as well as a PA, we have revised the current national modifier AS to read as follows:

AS— Physician Assistant, Nurse Practitioner, or Clinical Nurse Specialist services for assistant-at-surgery. (80 percent of the lesser of either the actual charge or 85 percent of the assistant-at-surgery payment for physicians.)

HCFA did not issue a national modifier for assistant-at-surgery services provided by NPs and CNSs before January 1, 1999; however, Carriers instructed the NPs and CNSs to submit the AS modifier when performing as an assistant-at-surgery for dates of service prior to January 1, 1999. HCFA has revised the 1999 HCPCS to reflect required use of the AS modifier by NPs and CNSs. This revision was effective January 1, 1999. Therefore, as noted in the revised language for this modifier, PAs, NPs and CNSs must use the AS modifier when billing as assistant-at-surgery.

These instructions should be implemented through your current operating budget.

This Program Memorandum may be discarded after April 1, 2000.

Contractors should address any questions to their appropriate regional office.

Appendix C.3

Program Memorandum B-98-47
Discontinuing the Surrogate Unique Physician Identification Number (UPIN) NPP000 for Nurse Practitioners (NPs), Clinical Nurse Specialists (CNSs), and Physician Assistants (PAs)

Document No. B-98-47 — Discontinuing the Surrogate Unique Physician Identification Number (UPIN) NPP000 for Nurse Practitioners (NPs), Clinical Nurse Specialists (CNSs), and Physician Assistants (PAs)

PROGRAM MEMORANDUM
CARRIERS
Department of Health and Human Services
Health Care Financing Administration
Transmittal No. B-98-47
Date: NOVEMBER 1998

Change Request #660

SUBJECT: Discontinuing the Surrogate Unique Physician Identification Number (UPIN) NPP000 for Nurse Practitioners (NPs), Clinical Nurse Specialists (CNSs), and Physician Assistants (PAs)

Effective January 1, 1998, [4511] §§4511 and [4512] 4512 of the Balanced Budget Act of 1997 removed the restrictions on the type of areas and settings in which the professional services of NPs, CNSs, and PAs are paid by Medicare. Accordingly, payments are allowed for services furnished by these non-physician practitioners in all areas and settings permitted under applicable State licensure laws. However, the provision maintains the current policy that no separate payment may be made to one of these non-physician practitioners when a facility or other provider payment or charge is also made for such professional services. (Refer to Program Memorandum AB-98-15, dated April 1998.)

The purpose of this program memorandum is to announce that HCFA is discontinuing the use of the surrogate UPIN "NPP000"effective January 1, 1999. "NPP000" has been used by NPs, CNSs, and PAs, because a permanent UPIN had not been issued to them. A mass mailing of letters containing language generated from HCFA Central Office and permanent UPINs for all NPs/CNSs/PAs, who are currently enrolled as Medicare providers, will be sent from Transamerica Occidental Life Insurance Company shortly. These non-physician practitioners should begin using their permanent UPINs immediately. You must issue a permanent UPIN to any new NP/CNS/PA who is applying to become a Medicare provider. In the future, as systems changes permit, claims containing the surrogate UPIN "NPP000" will be returned as unprocessable.

Physicians and non-physician providers who order or refer services must submit their names and their UPINs on Form HCFA-1500. This information must appear in block 17 and 17a of Form HCFA- 1500. For National Standard Format claims, the UPIN must appear in record/field FB1-09.0 as the ordering/referring provider. Providers submitting American National Standards Institute claims must submit a UPIN in X12N837 field:2-500.E-NM109.

Services of a NP or a CNS who is working in collaboration with, but independent of, a physician would be considered covered services as defined in [1861(s)(1)] §§ 1861(s)(l) and [1861(s)(2)(A)] 1861(s)(2)(A). Therefore, a NP or CNS who is treating the beneficiary can order or prescribe items of durable medical equipment, orthotics, prosthetics, and supplies (DMEPOS) and can complete Section D of the Certificate of Medical Necessity (CMN) if he or she is permitted to prescribe items of DMEPOS by the State in which the services were rendered. The NP and CNS must bill using their own provider number, and they must attest, the same as a physician, that they have treated the beneficiary and that all information presented in Section B of the CMN, or on the order, is true, accurate, and complete to the best of their knowledge. The name and UPIN of the NP or CNS are required on the CMN.

The Medicare Carriers Manual, Part 4, § 1009 will be updated to reflect this change.

HCFA-Pub. 60B

NPs, CNSs, and PAs need to be educated on how to use their permanent UPINs and not to use the surrogate UPIN "NPP000" for dates of services on or after January 1, 1999.

These instructions should be implemented within your current operating budget.

Questions regarding UPINs can be directed to Gerald Wright at (410)786-5798. Part B operational billing questions can be directed to Patricia Gill at (410)786-1297 and DMERC billing questions can be directed to Joanne Spalding on (410)786-3352.

This Program Memorandum may be discarded November 1999.

Appendix C.4

Program Memorandum B-00-2
Payment for Teleconsultations in Rural Health Professional Shortage Areas [January 1, 2000]

Document No. B-00-2 — Payment for Teleconsultations in Rural Health Professional Shortage Areas [January 1, 2000]

PROGRAM MEMORANDUM
CARRIERS
Department of Health and Human Services
Health Care Financing Administration
Transmittal No. B-99-02
Date: JANUARY 2000

This Program Memorandum re-issues Program Memorandum B-99-2, Change Request 545 dated January 1999. The only change is the discard date; all other material remains the same.

CHANGE REQUEST #545

SUBJECT: Payment for Teleconsultations in Rural Health Professional Shortage Areas

This program memorandum (PM) contains billing instructions for carriers to use in processing claims from physicians and other practitioners who furnish teleconsultations to Medicare beneficiaries who reside in a rural area designated as a health professional shortage area (HPSA). Carriers must begin processing claims for teleconsultations April 1, 1999 for dates of service January 1, 1999 and later.

Background

Section 4206 of the Balanced Budget Act (BBA) of 1997 provides coverage and payment for professional consultations with physicians and certain other practitioners via telecommunication systems. Payment may be made if the physician or other practitioner is furnishing a consultation via a telecommunication system to a beneficiary who resides in a rural area designated as a HPSA. The term practitioner will be used hereafter to include both physicians and non-physician practitioners.

Teleconsultation typically involves a primary care practitioner with a patient at a remote, rural (spoke) site and a medical specialist (consultant) at an urban or referral center (hub) facility, with the primary care practitioner seeking advice from the consultant concerning the patient's condition or course of treatment.

The BBA requires that Medicare Part B (Supplementary Medical Insurance) pay for professional consultation via telecommunication systems by January 1, 1999. Consultations rendered in this manner are titled teleconsultations. Teleconsultations apply to consultations for rural beneficiaries whether or not the consultant and primary care practitioner are located in the same area.

Definition of Professional Consultation Services Via Telecommunications Systems

A teleconsultation must be an interactive patient encounter that meets the criteria in the Physician's Current Procedural Terminology (CPT) descriptor for a given consultation service and includes the following:

■ Clinical assessment via medical examination directed by the consultant (specialist);

■ The use of audiovisual communications equipment that permits real time communication among the beneficiary, the consultant and the presenting practitioner.

NOTE: It is permissible for another practitioner to present the patient in lieu of the referring practitioner. However, if a practitioner other than the actual referring practitioner presents the patient, he or she must be an employee of the referring practitioner.

HCFA-Pub. 60B

■ Participation of a referring practitioner as appropriate to the medical needs of the patient, and as needed to provide information to and at the direction of the consultant; and

■ Feedback of the consultation assessment to the referring practitioner.

The above telecommunications requirements do not mandate the use of full motion video. If the telecommunications technology permits two way interactive audio and video communications that allow the consultant practitioner to conduct a medical exam, Medicare may make payment for a teleconsultation. For Medicare payment to be made, the patient must be present and the telecommunications technology must allow the consultant to conduct a medical examination of the patient.

The requirements do not prohibit the use of higher end store and forward technology in which less than full motion video is sufficient to perform an interactive examination at the control of the consultant. When performed in real time, with the patient present, store and forward may allow the consulting practitioner to control the examination by requesting additional, real time pictures of the patient that are transmitted immediately to the on-line consultant.

Payment Limitations

Section 4206 of the BBA provides that the amount of reimbursement for the teleconsultation may not exceed the amount in the current fee schedule applicable to the consulting practitioner's services. The payment may not include reimbursement for telephone line charges or any facility fees. Teleconsultations are subject to the coinsurance and deductible requirements under §1833(a)(1) and 1833 (b) of the Social Security Act.

Provider Submission of Claims for Teleconsultation

Claims for teleconsultations for dates of service January 1, 1999 and later must be submitted with the appropriate CPT code and the teleconsultation modifier "GT - Via Interactive Audio and Video Telecommunication Systems." By using the modifier to bill for the consultation, the consulting practitioner has authenticated that an eligible practitioner has served as the referring practitioner (See section "Providers Who May Bill for a Teleconsultation").

Reimbursement for a Teleconsultation

Medicare payment for the services of the consultant and for the services of the referring practitioner are bundled. The consultant must remit 25 percent of the payment received for the teleconsultation to the referring practitioner.

Providers Who May Bill for a Teleconsultation

Only the consulting practitioner may bill for teleconsultation. Carriers may process claims for teleconsultations from the following types of providers:

- Physicians

- Physician assistants (through their employers)

- Nurse practitioners

- Clinical nurse specialists and

- Nurse midwives.

Referring practitioners may be any of the following:

- Physicians

- Physician assistants

- Nurse practitioners

- Clinical nurse specialists

- Nurse midwives

- Clinical psychologists and

- Clinical social workers.

Remittance Advice Messages

Providers who bill for teleconsultations for dates of service January 1, 1999 and later must be directed to share the payment amount received with the referring practitioner. For claims submitted to CWF that are approved for payment, contractors will use claim line level remark code M109 "We have provided you with a bundled payment for a teleconsultation. You must send twenty-five percent of this payment to the referring practitioner."

Carrier Provider Bulletin

Carriers must issue a provider bulletin announcing our new coverage policy for teleconsultations. In your next regularly scheduled bulletin issue the following bulletin:

"Medicare Payment for Teleconsultation in Rural Health Professional Shortage Areas (HPSAs)

HCFA provides Medicare payment for a teleconsultation in rural health professional shortage areas. Payment for teleconsultations represents a departure from traditional Medicare policy by allowing payment for a service which has historically required a face-to-face, "hands on" encounter. A summary of the provisions is outlined below.

Eligibility for Teleconsultation

Medicare beneficiaries residing in rural HPSAs are eligible to receive teleconsultation services. The site of presentation is a proxy for beneficiary residence. Teleconsultation may be provided in full and partial county HPSAs designated by section 332(a)(1)(A) of the Public Health Service Act.

Scope of Coverage

Covered services include initial, follow-up, or confirming consultations in hospitals, outpatient facilities, or medical offices delivered via interactive audio and video telecommunications systems (CPTcodes 99241-99245, 99251-99255, 99261-99263, and 99271-99275).

Practitioners Eligible to be Consulting and Referring Practitioners

Clinical psychologists, clinical social workers, certified registered nurse anesthetists, and anesthesiologist assistants do not provide consultation services payable under Medicare and therefore cannot provide a teleconsultation under this provision. Additionally, certified nurse anesthetists and anesthesiologist assistants are not eligible to be referring practitioners for a teleconsultation. Practitioners who may provide teleconsultations include the following: physicians, physician assistants, nurse practitioners, clinical nurse specialists, and nurse-midwives. Practitioners who may refer patients for teleconsultation include the following: physicians, physician assistants, nurse practitioners, clinical nurse specialists, nurse-midwives, clinical psychologists, and clinical social workers.

Conditions of Payment

The patient must be present at the time of consultation, the medical examination of the patient must be under the control of the consulting practitioner, and the consultation must take place via an interactive audio and video telecommunications system. Interactive telecommunications systems must be multi-media communications that, at a minimum, include audio and video equipment permitting real-time consultation among the patient, consulting practitioner, and referring practitioner (as appropriate). Telephones, facsimile machines, and electronic mail systems do not meet the requirements of interactive telecommunications systems.

The teleconsultation involves the participation of the referring practitioner or a practitioner eligible to be a referring practitioner who is an employee of the actual referring practitioner as appropriate to the medical needs of the beneficiary and to provide information to and at the direction of the consultant.

If the medical needs of the beneficiary do not necessitate the participation of a referring or presenting practitioner for all or a portion of a teleconsultation, we would not require a referring or presenting practitioner as a condition of payment.

However, we believe that the number of teleconsultations in which a referring or presenting practitioner would not be medically appropriate for at least a portion of the teleconsultation should be few. As noted above, the participation of a referring or presenting practitioner, use of interactive audio and video technology and the patient's real time presence are required as conditions of payment. These requirements are intended to serve as a reasonable substitute for a face-to-face examination which is a requirement for consultation under Medicare. The absence of a referring or presenting practitioner for the entire teleconsultation is subject to review.

Registered nurses and other medical professionals not included within the definition of a practitioner in section [1842(b)(18)(C)] 1842(b)(18)(C) of the Act are not permitted to act as presenters during teleconsultations.

Medicare Payment Policy

A single payment will be made to the consulting practitioner. The amount will equal the consultant's current fee schedule payment for a face-to-face consultation. The statute requires that the fee be shared by the referring and consulting practitioners. The consulting practitioner receives 75 percent, and the referring practitioner 25 percent, of the consulting practitioner's Medicare fee. The patient continues to be responsible for the 20-percent Medicare coinsurance.

Billing for Teleconsultation

The consulting practitioner will submit one claim for the consultation service and will provide the referring practitioner with 25 percent of any payment, including any deductible or coinsurance received for the consultation. A modifier will be used to identify the claim as a teleconsultation. Providers must submit the claim with the modifier "GT - via interactive audio and video telecommunication systems." The referring practitioner cannot submit a Medicare claim for the teleconsultation.

Carriers must issue this entire provider bulletin as it is stated in this document. No revisions may be made to delete any of the information contained in this bulletin. However, contractors may add additional information to the article as deemed necessary.

These instructions should be implemented within your current operating budget.

This PM may be discarded July 31, 2001.

All contractors should address questions or issues surrounding implementation of these instructions to their regional office contact. Regional Office staff should contact Joan Proctor- Young at (410) 786-0949 to resolve any questions or issues surrounding the processing of these claims.

Appendix C.5

HCFA Program Manual Transmittals

2050. SERVICES AND SUPPLIES

Services and supplies (including drugs and biologicals which cannot be self-administered) are those furnished incident to a physician's professional services. (Certain hospital services may also be covered as incident to physicians' services when rendered to hospital outpatients. Payment for these services is made under Part B to a hospital by the hospital's intermediary.)

To be covered incident to the services of a physician, services and supplies must be:

■ An integral, although incidental, part of the physician's professional service (see §2050.1);

■ Commonly rendered without charge or included in the physician's bill (see §2050.1A);

■ Of a type that are commonly furnished in physician's offices or clinics (see §2050.1A);

■ Furnished under the physician's direct personal supervision (see §2050.1B); and

■ Furnished by the physician or by an individual who qualifies as an employee of the physician. (See §2050.1C.)

2050.1 Incident to Physician's Professional Services.

Incident to a physician's professional services means that the services or supplies are furnished as an integral, although incidental, part of the physician's personal professional services in the course of diagnosis or treatment of an injury or illness.

A. Commonly Furnished in Physicians' Offices

Services and supplies commonly furnished in physicians' offices are covered under the incident to provision. Where supplies are clearly of a type a physician is not expected to have on hand in his/her office or where services are of a type not considered medically appropriate to provide in the office setting, they would not be covered under the incident to provision.

Supplies usually furnished by the physician in the course of performing his/her services, e.g., gauze, ointments, bandages, and oxygen, are also covered. Charges for such services and supplies must be included in the physicians' bills. (See §2049 regarding coverage of drugs and biologicals under this provision.) To be covered, supplies, including drugs and biologicals, must represent an expense to the physician. For example, where a patient purchases a drug and the physician administers it, the cost of the drug is not covered.

B. Direct Personal Supervision

Coverage of services and supplies incident to the professional services of a physician in private practice is limited to situations in which there is direct personal physician supervision. This applies to services of auxiliary personnel employed by the physician and working under his/her supervision, such as nurses, nonphysician anesthetists, psychologists, technicians, therapists, including physical therapists, and other aides. Thus, where a physician employs auxiliary personnel to assist him/her in rendering services to patients and includes the charges for their services in his/her own bills, the services of such personnel are considered incident to the physician's service if there is a physician's service rendered to which the services of such personnel are an incidental part and there is direct personal supervision by the physician.

This does not mean, however, that to be considered incident to each occasion of service by a nonphysician (or the furnishing of a supply) need also always be the occasion of the actual rendition of a personal professional service by the physician. Such a service or supply could be considered to be incident to when furnished during a course of treatment where the physician performs an initial service and subsequent services of a frequency which reflect his/her active participation in and management of the course of treatment. (However, the direct personal supervision requirement must still be met with respect to every nonphysician service.)

Direct personal supervision in the office setting does not mean that the physician must be present in the same room with his or her aide. However, the physician must be present in the office suite and immediately available to provide assistance and direction throughout the time the aide is performing services.

If auxiliary personnel perform services outside the office setting, e.g., in a patient's home or in an institution, their services are covered incident to a physician's service only if there is direct personal supervision by the physician. For example, if a nurse accompanied the physician on house calls and administered an injection, the nurse's services are covered. If the same nurse made the calls alone and administered the injection, the services are not covered (even when billed by the physician) since the physician is not providing direct personal supervision. Services provided by auxiliary personnel in an institution (e.g., skilled nursing facility, nursing, or convalescent home) present a special problem in determining whether direct physician supervision exists. The availability of the physician by telephone and the presence of the physician somewhere in the institution does not constitute direct personal supervision. (See §45-15 of the Coverage Issues Manual for instructions used if a physician maintains an office in an institution.) For hospital patients, there is no Medicare coverage of the services of physician-employed auxiliary personnel as services incident to physicians' services under §1861(s)(2)(A) of the Social Security Act. Such services can be covered only under the hospital outpatient or inpatient benefit and payment for such services can be made to only the hospital by a Medicare intermediary. For services in a hospital, see §2390. (See §2070 concerning physician supervision of technicians performing diagnostic X-ray procedures in a physician's office.)

C. Employment

To be considered an employee for purposes of this section, the nonphysician performing an incident to service may be a part-time, full-time, or leased employee of the supervising physician, physician group practice, or of the legal entity that employs the physician (hereafter referred to collectively as the physician or other entity) who provides direct personal supervision (as described below). A leased employee is a nonphysician working under a written employee leasing agreement which provides that:

- The nonphysician, although employed by the leasing company, provides services as the leased employee of the physician or other entity; and

- The physician or other entity exercises control over all actions taken by the leased employee with regard to the rendering of medical services to the same extent as the physician or other entity would exercise such control if the leased employee were directly employed by the physician or other entity.

In order to satisfy the employment requirement, the nonphysician (either leased or directly employed) must be considered an employee of the supervising physician or other entity under the common law test of an employer/employee relationship specified in 210(j)(2) of the Act, CFR 20 CFR 404.1007, and §RS 2101.020 of the Retirement and Survivors Insurance part of the Social Security Program Operations Manual System.

Services provided by auxiliary personnel not in the employ of the physician, physician group practice, or other legal entity, even if provided on the physician's order or included in the physician's bill are not covered as incident to a physician's service since the law requires that the services be of kinds commonly furnished in physicians' offices and commonly either rendered without charge or included in physicians' bills. As with the physicians' personal professional service, the patient's financial liability for the incidental services is to the physician, physician group practice, or other legal entity. Therefore, the incidental service must represent an expense incurred by the physician, physician group practice, or other legal entity responsible for providing the professional service.

2050.2 Services of Nonphysician Personnel Furnished Incident to Physician's Services.

In addition to coverage being available for the services of such nonphysician personnel as nurses, technicians, and therapists when furnished incident to the professional services of a physician (as discussed in §2050.1), a physician may also have the services of certain nonphysician practitioners covered as services incident to a physician's professional services. These nonphysician practitioners, who are being licensed by the States under various programs to assist or act in the place of the physician, include, for example, certified nurse midwives, certified registered nurse anesthetists, clinical psychologists, clinical social workers, physician assistants, nurse practitioners, and clinical nurse specialists. (See §§2150 through 2160 for coverage instructions for various allied health/nonphysician practitioners' services.)

Services performed by these nonphysician practitioners incident to a physician's professional services include not only services ordinarily rendered by a physician's office staff person (e.g., medical services such as taking blood pressures and temperatures, giving injections, and changing dressings) but also services ordinarily performed by the physician himself or herself such as minor surgery, setting casts or simple fractures, reading x-rays, and other activities that involve evaluation or treatment of a patient's condition.

Nonetheless, in order for services of a nonphysician practitioner to be covered as incident to the services of a physician, the services must meet all of the requirements for coverage specified in §§2050 through 2050.1. For example, the services must be an integral, although incidental, part of the physician's personal professional services, and they must be performed under the physician's direct personal supervision.

A nonphysician practitioner such as a physician assistant or a nurse practitioner may be licensed under State law to perform a specific medical procedure and may be able (see §§2156 or 2158, respectively) to perform the procedure without physician supervision and have the service separately covered and paid for by Medicare as a physician assistant or nurse practitioner service. However, in order to have that same service covered as incident to the services of a physician, it must be performed under the direct personal supervision of the physician of the physician as an integral part of the physician personal in-office service. As explained in §2050.1, this does not mean that each occasion of an incidental service performed by a nonphysician practitioner must always be the occasion of a service actually rendered by the physician. It does mean that there must have been a direct, personal, professional service furnished by the physician to initiate the course of treatment of which the service being performed by the nonphysician practitioner is an incidental part, and there must be subsequent services by the physician of a frequency that reflects his or her continuing active participation in and management of the course of treatment. In addition, the physician must be physically present in the same office suite and be immediately available to render assistance if that becomes necessary.

Note also that a physician might render a physician's service that can be covered even though another service furnished by a nonphysician practitioner as incident to the physician's service might not be covered. For example, an office visit during which the physician diagnoses a medical problem and established a course of treatment could be covered even if, during the same visit, a nonphysician practitioner performs a noncovered service such as an acupuncture.

2050.3 Incident to Physician's Service in Clinic.

Services and supplies incident to a physician's service in a physician directed clinic or group association are generally the same as those described above.

A physician directed clinic is one where (a) a physician (or a number of physicians) is present to perform medical (rather than administrative) services at all times the clinic is open; (b) each patient is under the care of a clinic physician; and (c) the nonphysician services are under medical supervision.

In highly organized clinics, particularly those that are departmentalized, direct personal physician supervision may be the responsibility of several physicians as opposed to an individual attending physician. In this situation, medical management of all services provided in the clinic is assured. The physician ordering a particular service need not be the physician who is supervising the service. Therefore, services performed by therapists and other aided are covered even though they are performed in another department of the clinic.

Supplies provided by the clinic during the course of treatment are also covered. When the auxiliary personnel perform services outside the clinic premises, the services are covered only if performed under the direct personal supervision of a clinic physician. If the clinic refers a patient for auxiliary services performed by personnel who are not employed by the clinic, such services are not incident to a physician's service.

Appendix D

AMA/HCFA

1997 and 1995 Documentation Guidelines for Evaluation and Management Services

1997 Documentation Guidelines for Evaluation and Management Services

This is an update of the guidelines jointly produced by the American Medical Association (AMA) and HCFA in May, 1997. It incorporates revisions to the gastrointestinal section of the general multi-system exam and the skin section of the single organ system exam of the skin. These revisions were approved by the AMA and HCFA in November, 1997.

American Medical Association
Health Care Financing Administration
November, 1997

Source: *Documentation Guidelines for Evaluation and Management Services,* ©1997. American Medical Association, *http://www.hcfa.gov/medicare/mcarpti.htm*

1997 Documentation Guidelines for Evaluation and Management Services

TABLE OF CONTENTS

1997 DOCUMENTATION GUIDELINES
FOR EVALUATION AND MANAGEMENT SERVICES

I.   **INTRODUCTION**

WHAT IS DOCUMENTATION AND WHY IS IT IMPORTANT?

Medical record documentation is required to record pertinent facts, findings, and observations about an individual's health history including past and present illnesses, examinations, tests, treatments, and outcomes. The medical record chronologically documents the care of the patient and is an important element contributing to high quality care. The medical record facilitates:

- the ability of the physician and other health care professionals to evaluate and plan the patient's immediate treatment, and to monitor his/her health care over time.

- communication and continuity of care among physicians and other health care professionals involved in the patient's care;

- accurate and timely claims review and payment;

- appropriate utilization review and quality of care evaluations; and

- collection of data that may be useful for research and education.

An appropriately documented medical record can reduce many of the "hassles" associated with claims processing and may serve as a legal document to verify the care provided, if necessary.

WHAT DO PAYERS WANT AND WHY?

Because payers have a contractual obligation to enrollees, they may require reasonable documentation that services are consistent with the insurance coverage provided. They may request information to validate:

- the site of service;

- the medical necessity and appropriateness of the diagnostic and/or therapeutic services provided; and/or

- that services provided have been accurately reported.

II. GENERAL PRINCIPLES OF MEDICAL RECORD DOCUMENTATION

The principles of documentation listed below are applicable to all types of medical and surgical services in all settings. For Evaluation and Management (E/M) services, the nature and amount of physician work and documentation varies by type of service, place of service and the patient's status. The general principles listed below may be modified to account for these variable circumstances in providing E/M services.

1. The medical record should be complete and legible.

2. The documentation of each patient encounter should include:

   - reason for the encounter and relevant history, physical examination findings and prior diagnostic test results;

   - assessment, clinical impression or diagnosis;

   - plan for care; and

   - date and legible identity of the observer.

3. If not documented, the rationale for ordering diagnostic and other ancillary services should be easily inferred.

4. Past and present diagnoses should be accessible to the treating and/or consulting physician.

5. Appropriate health risk factors should be identified.

6. The patient's progress, response to and changes in treatment, and revision of diagnosis should be documented.

7. The CPT and ICD-9-CM codes reported on the health insurance claim form or billing statement should be supported by the documentation in the medical record.

III. DOCUMENTATION OF E/M SERVICES

This publication provides definitions and documentation guidelines for the three key components of E/M services and for visits which consist predominately of counseling or coordination of care. The three *key* components--history, examination, and medical decision making--appear in the descriptors for office and other outpatient services, hospital observation services, hospital inpatient services, consultations, emergency department services, nursing facility services, domiciliary care services, and home services. While some of the text of CPT has been repeated in this publication, the reader should refer to CPT for the complete descriptors for E/M services and instructions for selecting a level of service. Documentation guidelines are identified by the symbol •*DG*.

The descriptors for the levels of E/M services recognize seven components which are used in defining the levels of E/M services. These components are:

- history;
- examination;
- medical decision making;
- counseling;
- coordination of care;
- nature of presenting problem; and
- time.

The first three of these components (i.e., history, examination and medical decision making) are the key components in selecting the level of E/M services. In the case of visits which consist <u>predominantly</u> of counseling or coordination of care, time is the key or controlling factor to qualify for a particular level of E/M service.

Because the level of E/M service is dependent on two or three key components, performance and documentation of one component (eg, examination) at the highest level does not necessarily mean that the encounter in its entirety qualifies for the highest level of E/M service.

These Documentation Guidelines for E/M services reflect the needs of the typical adult population. For certain groups of patients, the recorded information may vary slightly from that described here. Specifically, the medical records of infants, children, adolescents and pregnant women may have additional or modified information recorded in each history and examination area.

As an example, newborn records may include under history of the present illness (HPI) the details of mother's pregnancy and the infant's status at birth; social history will focus on family structure; family history will focus on congenital

4

anomalies and hereditary disorders in the family. In addition, the content of a pediatric examination will vary with the age and development of the child. Although not specifically defined in these documentation guidelines, these patient group variations on history and examination are appropriate.

A. DOCUMENTATION OF HISTORY

The levels of E/M services are based on four types of history (Problem Focused, Expanded Problem Focused, Detailed, and Comprehensive). Each type of history includes some or all of the following elements:

- Chief complaint (CC);

- History of present illness (HPI);

- Review of systems (ROS); and

- Past, family and/or social history (PFSH).

The extent of history of present illness, review of systems and past, family and/or social history that is obtained and documented is dependent upon clinical judgement and the nature of the presenting problem(s).

The chart below shows the progression of the elements required for each type of history. To qualify for a given type of history all three elements in the table must be met. (A chief complaint is indicated at all levels.)

History of Present Illness (HPI)	Review of Systems (ROS)	Past, Family, and/or Social History (PFSH)	Type of History
Brief	N/A	N/A	*Problem Focused*
Brief	Problem Pertinent	N/A	*Expanded Problem Focused*
Extended	Extended	Pertinent	*Detailed*
Extended	Complete	Complete	*Comprehensive*

●*DG:* *The CC, ROS and PFSH may be listed as separate elements of history, or they may be included in the description of the history of the present illness.*

●*DG:* *A ROS and/or a PFSH obtained during an earlier encounter does not need to be re-recorded if there is evidence that the physician reviewed and updated the previous information. This may occur when a physician updates his or her own record or in an institutional setting or group practice where many physicians use a common record. The review and update may be documented by:*

- *describing any new ROS and/or PFSH information or noting there has been no change in the information; and*

- *noting the date and location of the earlier ROS and/or PFSH.*

●*DG:* *The ROS and/or PFSH may be recorded by ancillary staff or on a form completed by the patient. To document that the physician reviewed the information, there must be a notation supplementing or confirming the information recorded by others.*

●*DG:* *If the physician is unable to obtain a history from the patient or other source, the record should describe the patient's condition or other circumstance which precludes obtaining a history.*

Definitions and specific documentation guidelines for each of the elements of history are listed below.

CHIEF COMPLAINT (CC)

The CC is a concise statement describing the symptom, problem, condition, diagnosis, physician recommended return, or other factor that is the reason for the encounter, usually stated in the patient's words.

●*DG:* *The medical record should clearly reflect the chief complaint.*

HISTORY OF PRESENT ILLNESS (HPI)

The HPI is a chronological description of the development of the patient's present illness from the first sign and/or symptom or from the previous encounter to the present. It includes the following elements:

- location,
- quality,
- severity,
- duration,
- timing,
- context,
- modifying factors, and
- associated signs and symptoms.

Brief and *extended* HPIs are distinguished by the amount of detail needed to accurately characterize the clinical problem(s).

A *brief* HPI consists of one to three elements of the HPI.

> ●*DG: The medical record should describe one to three elements of the present illness (HPI).*

An *extended* HPI consists of at least four elements of the HPI or the status of at least three chronic or inactive conditions.

> ●*DG: The medical record should describe at least four elements of the present illness (HPI), or the status of at least three chronic or inactive conditions.*

REVIEW OF SYSTEMS (ROS)

A ROS is an inventory of body systems obtained through a series of questions seeking to identify signs and/or symptoms which the patient may be experiencing or has experienced.

For purposes of ROS, the following systems are recognized:

- Constitutional symptoms (e.g., fever, weight loss)
- Eyes
- Ears, Nose, Mouth, Throat
- Cardiovascular
- Respiratory
- Gastrointestinal
- Genitourinary
- Musculoskeletal
- Integumentary (skin and/or breast)
- Neurological
- Psychiatric
- Endocrine
- Hematologic/Lymphatic
- Allergic/Immunologic

A *problem pertinent* ROS inquires about the system directly related to the problem(s) identified in the HPI.

> ●*DG: The patient's positive responses and pertinent negatives for the system related to the problem should be documented.*

An *extended* ROS inquires about the system directly related to the problem(s) identified in the HPI and a limited number of additional systems.

> ●*DG: The patient's positive responses and pertinent negatives for two to nine systems should be documented.*

A *complete* ROS inquires about the system(s) directly related to the problem(s) identified in the HPI *plus* all additional body systems.

> ●*DG: At least ten organ systems must be reviewed. Those systems with positive or pertinent negative responses must be individually documented. For the remaining systems, a notation indicating all other systems are negative is permissible. In the absence of such a notation, at least ten systems must be individually documented.*

PAST, FAMILY AND/OR SOCIAL HISTORY (PFSH)

The PFSH consists of a review of three areas:

- past history (the patient's past experiences with illnesses, operations, injuries and treatments);

- family history (a review of medical events in the patient's family, including diseases which may be hereditary or place the patient at risk); and

- social history (an age appropriate review of past and current activities).

For certain categories of E/M services that include only an interval history, it is not necessary to record information about the PFSH. Those categories are subsequent hospital care, follow-up inpatient consultations and subsequent nursing facility care.

A *pertinent* PFSH is a review of the history area(s) directly related to the problem(s) identified in the HPI.

> ●DG: *At least one specific item from any of the three history areas must be documented for a pertinent PFSH .*

A *complete* PFSH is of a review of two or all three of the PFSH history areas, depending on the category of the E/M service. A review of all three history areas is required for services that by their nature include a comprehensive assessment or reassessment of the patient. A review of two of the three history areas is sufficient for other services.

> ●DG: *At least one specific item from two of the three history areas must be documented for a complete PFSH for the following categories of E/M services: office or other outpatient services, established patient; emergency department; domiciliary care, established patient; and home care, established patient.*

> ●DG: *At least one specific item from each of the three history areas must be documented for a complete PFSH for the following categories of E/M services: office or other outpatient services, new patient; hospital observation services; hospital inpatient services, initial care; consultations; comprehensive nursing facility assessments; domiciliary care, new patient; and home care, new patient.*

B. DOCUMENTATION OF EXAMINATION

The levels of E/M services are based on four types of examination:

- *Problem Focused* -- a limited examination of the affected body area or organ system.

- *Expanded Problem Focused* -- a limited examination of the affected body area or organ system and any ther symptomatic or related body area(s) or organ system(s).

- *Detailed* -- an extended examination of the affected body area(s) or organ system(s) and any other symptomatic or related body area(s) or organ system(s).

- *Comprehensive* -- a general multi-system examination, or complete examination of a single organ system and other symptomatic or related body area(s) or organ system(s).

These types of examinations have been defined for general multi-system and the following single organ systems:

- Cardiovascular
- Ears, Nose, Mouth and Throat
- Eyes
- Genitourinary (Female)
- Genitourinary (Male)
- Hematologic/Lymphatic/Immunologic
- Musculoskeletal
- Neurological
- Psychiatric
- Respiratory
- Skin

A general multi-system examination or a single organ system examination may be performed by any physician regardless of specialty. The type (general multi-system or single organ system) and content of examination are selected by the examining physician and are based upon clinical judgement, the patient's history, and the nature of the presenting problem(s).

The content and documentation requirements for each type and level of examination are summarized below and described in detail in tables beginning on page 13. In the tables, organ systems and body areas recognized by CPT for purposes of describing examinations are shown in the left column. The content, or individual elements, of the examination pertaining to that body area or organ system are identified by bullets (•) in the right column.

Parenthetical examples, "(eg, ...)", have been used for clarification and to provide guidance regarding documentation. Documentation for each element must satisfy any numeric requirements (such as "Measurement of *any three of the following seven...*") included in the description of the element. Elements with multiple components but with no specific numeric requirement (such as "Examination of *liver* and *spleen*") require documentation of at least one component. It is possible for a given examination to be expanded beyond what is defined here. When that occurs, findings related to the additional systems and/or areas should be documented.

> •*DG: Specific abnormal and relevant negative findings of the examination of the affected or symptomatic body area(s) or organ system(s) should be documented. A notation of "abnormal" without elaboration is insufficient.*
> •*DG: Abnormal or unexpected findings of the examination of any asymptomatic body area(s) or organ system(s) should be described.*
>
> •*DG: A brief statement or notation indicating "negative" or "normal" is sufficient to document normal findings related to unaffected area(s) or asymptomatic organ system(s).*

GENERAL MULTI-SYSTEM EXAMINATIONS

General multi-system examinations are described in detail beginning on page 13. To qualify for a given level of multi-system examination, the following content and documentation requirements should be met:

- *Problem Focused Examination*-should include performance and documentation of one to five elements identified by a bullet (•) in one or more organ system(s) or body area(s).

- *Expanded Problem Focused Examination*-should include performance and documentation of at least six elements identified by a bullet (•) in one or more organ system(s) or body area(s).

- *Detailed Examination*--should include at least six organ systems or body areas. For each system/area selected, performance and documentation of at least two elements identified by a bullet (•) is expected. Alternatively, a detailed examination may include performance and documentation of at least twelve elements identified by a bullet (•) in two or more organ systems or body areas.

- *Comprehensive Examination*--should include at least nine organ systems or body areas. For each system/area selected, all elements of the examination identified by a bullet (•) should be performed, unless specific directions limit the content of the examination. For each area/system, documentation of at least two elements identified by a bullet is expected.

SINGLE ORGAN SYSTEM EXAMINATIONS

The single organ system examinations recognized by CPT are described in detail beginning on page 18. Variations among these examinations in the organ systems and body areas identified in the left columns and in the elements of the examinations described in the right columns reflect differing emphases among specialties. To qualify for a given level of single organ system examination, the following content and documentation requirements should be met:

- *Problem Focused Examination*--should include performance and documentation of one to five elements identified by a bullet (•), whether in a box with a shaded or unshaded border.

- *Expanded Problem Focused Examination*--should include performance and documentation of at least six elements identified by a bullet (•), whether in a box with a shaded or unshaded border.

- *Detailed Examination*--examinations other than the eye and psychiatric examinations should include performance and documentation of at least twelve elements identified by a bullet (•), whether in box with a shaded or unshaded border.

    Eye and psychiatric examinations should include
    the performance and documentation of at least
    nine elements identified by a bullet (•), whether
    in a box with a shaded or unshaded border.

- *Comprehensive Examination*--should include performance of all elements identified by a bullet (•), whether in a shaded or unshaded box. Documentation of every element in each box with a shaded border and at least one element in each box with an unshaded border is expected.

12

CONTENT AND DOCUMENTATION REQUIREMENTS

General Multi-System Examination

System/Body Area	Elements of Examination
Constitutional	• Measurement of **any three of the following seven** vital signs: 1) sitting or standing blood pressure, 2) supine blood pressure, 3) pulse rate and regularity, 4) respiration, 5) temperature, 6) height, 7) weight (May be measured and recorded by ancillary staff) • General appearance of patient (eg, development, nutrition, body habitus, deformities, attention to grooming)
Eyes	• Inspection of conjunctivae and lids • Examination of pupils and irises (eg, reaction to light and accommodation, size and symmetry) • Ophthalmoscopic examination of optic discs (eg, size, C/D ratio, appearance) and posterior segments (eg, vessel changes, exudates, hemorrhages)
Ears, Nose, Mouth and Throat	• External inspection of ears and nose (eg, overall appearance, scars, lesions, masses) • Otoscopic examination of external auditory canals and tympanic membranes • Assessment of hearing (eg, whispered voice, finger rub, tuning fork) • Inspection of nasal mucosa, septum and turbinates • Inspection of lips, teeth and gums • Examination of oropharynx: oral mucosa, salivary glands, hard and soft palates, tongue, tonsils and posterior pharynx
Neck	• Examination of neck (eg, masses, overall appearance, symmetry, tracheal position, crepitus) • Examination of thyroid (eg, enlargement, tenderness, mass)

System/Body Area	Elements of Examination
Respiratory	• Assessment of respiratory effort (eg, intercostal retractions, use of accessory muscles, diaphragmatic movement) • Percussion of chest (eg, dullness, flatness, hyperresonance) • Palpation of chest (eg, tactile fremitus) • Auscultation of lungs (eg, breath sounds, adventitious sounds, rubs)
Cardiovascular	• Palpation of heart (eg, location, size, thrills) • Auscultation of heart with notation of abnormal sounds and murmurs Examination of: • carotid arteries (eg, pulse amplitude, bruits) • abdominal aorta (eg, size, bruits) • femoral arteries (eg, pulse amplitude, bruits) • pedal pulses (eg, pulse amplitude) • extremities for edema and/or varicosities
Chest (Breasts)	• Inspection of breasts (eg, symmetry, nipple discharge) • Palpation of breasts and axillae (eg, masses or lumps, tenderness)
Gastrointestinal (Abdomen)	• Examination of abdomen with notation of presence of masses or tenderness • Examination of liver and spleen • Examination for presence or absence of hernia • Examination (when indicated) of anus, perineum and rectum, including sphincter tone, presence of hemorrhoids, rectal masses • Obtain stool sample for occult blood test when indicated

System/Body Area	Elements of Examination
Genitourinary	**MALE:** • Examination of the scrotal contents (eg, hydrocele, spermatocele, tenderness of cord, testicular mass) • Examination of the penis • Digital rectal examination of prostate gland (eg, size, symmetry, nodularity, tenderness) **FEMALE:** Pelvic examination (with or without specimen collection for smears and cultures), including • Examination of external genitalia (eg, general appearance, hair distribution, lesions) and vagina (eg, general appearance, estrogen effect, discharge, lesions, pelvic support, cystocele, rectocele) • Examination of urethra (eg, masses, tenderness, scarring) • Examination of bladder (eg, fullness, masses, tenderness) • Cervix (eg, general appearance, lesions, discharge) • Uterus (eg, size, contour, position, mobility, tenderness, consistency, descent or support) • Adnexa/parametria (eg, masses, tenderness, organomegaly, nodularity)
Lymphatic	Palpation of lymph nodes in **two or more** areas: • Neck • Axillae • Groin • Other

System/Body Area	Elements of Examination
Musculoskeletal	• Examination of gait and station • Inspection and/or palpation of digits and nails (eg, clubbing, cyanosis, inflammatory conditions, petechiae, ischemia, infections, nodes) Examination of joints, bones and muscles of **one or more of the following six** areas: 1) head and neck; 2) spine, ribs and pelvis; 3) right upper extremity; 4) left upper extremity; 5) right lower extremity; and 6) left lower extremity. The examination of a given area includes: • Inspection and/or palpation with notation of presence of any misalignment, asymmetry, crepitation, defects, tenderness, masses, effusions • Assessment of range of motion with notation of any pain, crepitation or contracture • Assessment of stability with notation of any dislocation (luxation), subluxation or laxity • Assessment of muscle strength and tone (eg, flaccid, cog wheel, spastic) with notation of any atrophy or abnormal movements
Skin	• Inspection of skin and subcutaneous tissue (eg, rashes, lesions, ulcers) • Palpation of skin and subcutaneous tissue (eg, induration, subcutaneous nodules, tightening)
Neurologic	• Test cranial nerves with notation of any deficits • Examination of deep tendon reflexes with notation of pathological reflexes (eg, Babinski) • Examination of sensation (eg, by touch, pin, vibration, proprioception)
Psychiatric	• Description of patient's judgment and insight Brief assessment of mental status including: • orientation to time, place and person • recent and remote memory • mood and affect (eg, depression, anxiety, agitation)

Content and Documentation Requirements

Level of Exam	Perform and Document:
Problem Focused	**One to five** elements identified by a bullet.
Expanded Problem Focused	**At least six** elements identified by a bullet.
Detailed	**At least two** elements identified by a bullet **from each of six areas/systems** OR **at least twelve** elements identified by a bullet **in two or more areas/systems**.
Comprehensive	Perform **all elements** identified by a bullet in **at least nine** organ systems or body areas and document **at least two** elements identified by a bullet **from each of nine areas/systems**.

Cardiovascular Examination

System/Body Area	Elements of Examination
Constitutional	• Measurement of **any three of the following seven** vital signs: 1) sitting or standing blood pressure, 2) supine blood pressure, 3) pulse rate and regularity, 4) respiration, 5) temperature, 6) height, 7) weight (May be measured and recorded by ancillary staff) • General appearance of patient (eg, development, nutrition, body habitus, deformities, attention to grooming)
Head and Face	
Eyes	• Inspection of conjunctivae and lids (eg, xanthelasma)
Ears, Nose, Mouth and Throat	• Inspection of teeth, gums and palate • Inspection of oral mucosa with notation of presence of pallor or cyanosis
Neck	• Examination of jugular veins (eg, distension; a, v or cannon a waves) • Examination of thyroid (eg, enlargement, tenderness, mass)
Respiratory	• Assessment of respiratory effort (eg, intercostal retractions, use of accessory muscles, diaphragmatic movement) • Auscultation of lungs (eg, breath sounds, adventitious sounds, rubs)
Cardiovascular	• Palpation of heart (eg, location, size and forcefulness of the point of maximal impact; thrills; lifts; palpable S3 or S4) • Auscultation of heart including sounds, abnormal sounds and murmurs • Measurement of blood pressure in two or more extremities when indicated (eg, aortic dissection, coarctation) Examination of: • Carotid arteries (eg, waveform, pulse amplitude, bruits, apical-carotid delay) • Abdominal aorta (eg, size, bruits) • Femoral arteries (eg, pulse amplitude, bruits) • Pedal pulses (eg, pulse amplitude) • Extremities for peripheral edema and/or varicosities

System/Body Area	Elements of Examination
Chest (Breasts)	
Gastrointestinal (Abdomen)	• Examination of abdomen with notation of presence of masses or tenderness • Examination of liver and spleen • Obtain stool sample for occult blood from patients who are being considered for thrombolytic or anticoagulant therapy
Genitourinary (Abdomen)	
Lymphatic	
Musculoskeletal	• Examination of the back with notation of kyphosis or scoliosis • Examination of gait with notation of ability to undergo exercise testing and/or participation in exercise programs • Assessment of muscle strength and tone (eg, flaccid, cog wheel, spastic) with notation of any atrophy and abnormal movements
Extremities	• Inspection and palpation of digits and nails (eg, clubbing, cyanosis, inflammation, petechiae, ischemia, infections, Osler's nodes)
Skin	• Inspection and/or palpation of skin and subcutaneous tissue (eg, stasis dermatitis, ulcers, scars, xanthomas)
Neurological/ Psychiatric	Brief assessment of mental status including • Orientation to time, place and person, • Mood and affect (eg, depression, anxiety, agitation)

Content and Documentation Requirements

Level of Exam	Perform and Document:
Problem Focused	**One to five** elements identified by a bullet.
Expanded Problem Focused	**At least six** elements identified by a bullet.
Detailed	**At least twelve** elements identified by a bullet.
Comprehensive	Perform **all** elements identified by a bullet; document every element in each box with a shaded border and at least one element in each box with an unshaded border.

Ear, Nose and Throat Examination

System/Body Area	Elements of Examination
Constitutional	• Measurement of **any three of the following seven** vital signs: 1) sitting or standing blood pressure, 2) supine blood pressure, 3) pulse rate and regularity, 4) respiration, 5) temperature, 6) height, 7) weight (May be measured and recorded by ancillary staff) • General appearance of patient (eg, development, nutrition, body habitus, deformities, attention to grooming) • Assessment of ability to communicate (eg, use of sign language or other communication aids) and quality of voice
Head and Face	• Inspection of head and face (eg, overall appearance, scars, lesions and masses) • Palpation and/or percussion of face with notation of presence or absence of sinus tenderness • Examination of salivary glands • Assessment of facial strength
Eyes	• Test ocular motility including primary gaze alignment
Ears, Nose, Mouth and Throat	• Otoscopic examination of external auditory canals and tympanic membranes including pneumo-otoscopy with notation of mobility of membranes • Assessment of hearing with tuning forks and clinical speech reception thresholds (eg, whispered voice, finger rub) • External inspection of ears and nose (eg, overall appearance, scars, lesions and masses) • Inspection of nasal mucosa, septum and turbinates • Inspection of lips, teeth and gums • Examination of oropharynx: oral mucosa, hard and soft palates, tongue, tonsils and posterior pharynx (eg, asymmetry, lesions, hydration of mucosal surfaces) • Inspection of pharyngeal walls and pyriform sinuses (eg, pooling of saliva, asymmetry, lesions) • Examination by mirror of larynx including the condition of the epiglottis, false vocal cords, true vocal cords and mobility of larynx (Use of mirror not required in children) • Examination by mirror of nasopharynx including appearance of the mucosa, adenoids, posterior choanae and eustachian tubes (Use of mirror not required in children)

System/Body Area	Elements of Examination
Neck	• Examination of neck (eg, masses, overall appearance, symmetry, tracheal position, crepitus) • Examination of thyroid (eg, enlargement, tenderness, mass)
Respiratory	• Inspection of chest including symmetry, expansion and/or assessment of respiratory effort (eg, intercostal retractions, use of accessory muscles, diaphragmatic movement) • Auscultation of lungs (eg, breath sounds, adventitious sounds, rubs)
Cardiovascular	• Auscultation of heart with notation of abnormal sounds and murmurs • Examination of peripheral vascular system by observation (eg, swelling, varicosities) and palpation (eg, pulses, temperature, edema, tenderness)
Chest (Breasts)	
Gastrointestinal (Abdomen)	
Genitourinary	
Lymphatic	• Palpation of lymph nodes in neck, axillae, groin and/or other location
Musculoskeletal	
Extremities	
Skin	
Neurological/ Psychiatric	• Test cranial nerves with notation of any deficits Brief assessment of mental status including • Orientation to time, place and person, • Mood and affect (eg, depression, anxiety, agitation)

Content and Documentation Requirements

Level of Exam	Perform and Document:
Problem Focused	**One to five** elements identified by a bullet.
Expanded Problem Focused	**At least six** elements identified by a bullet.
Detailed	**At least twelve** elements identified by a bullet.
Comprehensive	Perform **all** elements identified by a bullet; document every element in each box with a shaded border and at least one element in each box with an unshaded border.

Eye Examination

System/Body Area	Elements of Examination
Constitutional	
Head and Face	
Eyes	• Test visual acuity (Does not include determination of refractive error) • Gross visual field testing by confrontation • Test ocular motility including primary gaze alignment • Inspection of bulbar and palpebral conjunctivae • Examination of ocular adnexae including lids (eg, ptosis or lagophthalmos), lacrimal glands, lacrimal drainage, orbits and preauricular lymph nodes • Examination of pupils and irises including shape, direct and consensual reaction (afferent pupil), size (eg, anisocoria) and morphology • Slit lamp examination of the corneas including epithelium, stroma, endothelium, and tear film • Slit lamp examination of the anterior chambers including depth, cells, and flare • Slit lamp examination of the lenses including clarity, anterior and posterior capsule, cortex, and nucleus • Measurement of intraocular pressures (except in children and patients with trauma or infectious disease) Ophthalmoscopic examination through dilated pupils (unless contraindicated) of • Optic discs including size, C/D ratio, appearance (eg, atrophy, cupping, tumor elevation) and nerve fiber layer • Posterior segments including retina and vessels (eg, exudates and hemorrhages)
Ears, Nose, Mouth and Throat	
Neck	
Respiratory	

System/Body Area	Elements of Examination
Cardiovascular	
Chest (Breasts)	
Gastrointestinal (Abdomen)	
Genitourinary	
Lymphatic	
Musculoskeletal	
Extremities	
Skin	
Neurological/ Psychiatric	Brief assessment of mental status including • Orientation to time, place and person • Mood and affect (eg, depression, anxiety, agitation)

Content and Documentation Requirements

Level of Exam	Perform and Document:
Problem Focused	**One to five** elements identified by a bullet.
Expanded Problem Focused	**At least six** elements identified by a bullet.
Detailed	**At least nine** elements identified by a bullet.
Comprehensive	Perform **all** elements identified by a bullet; document every element in each box with a shaded border and at least one element in each box with an unshaded border.

Genitourinary Examination

System/Body Area	Elements of Examination
Constitutional	• Measurement of **any three of the following seven** vital signs: 1) sitting or standing blood pressure, 2) supine blood pressure, 3) pulse rate and regularity, 4) respiration, 5) temperature, 6) height, 7) weight (May be measured and recorded by ancillary staff) • General appearance of patient (eg, development, nutrition, body habitus, deformities, attention to grooming)
Head and Face	
Eyes	
Ears, Nose, Mouth and Throat	
Neck	• Examination of neck (eg, masses, overall appearance, symmetry, tracheal position, crepitus) • Examination of thyroid (eg, enlargement, tenderness, mass)
Respiratory	• Assessment of respiratory effort (eg, intercostal retractions, use of accessory muscles, diaphragmatic movement) • Auscultation of lungs (eg, breath sounds, adventitious sounds, rubs)
Cardiovascular	• Auscultation of heart with notation of abnormal sounds and murmurs • Examination of peripheral vascular system by observation (eg, swelling, varicosities) and palpation (eg, pulses, temperature, edema, tenderness)
Chest (Breasts)	[See genitourinary (female)]
Gastrointestinal (Abdomen)	• Examination of abdomen with notation of presence of masses or tenderness • Examination for presence or absence of hernia • Examination of liver and spleen • Obtain stool sample for occult blood test when indicated

System/Body Area	Elements of Examination
Genitourinary	**MALE:** • Inspection of anus and perineum Examination (with or without specimen collection for smears and cultures) of genitalia including: • Scrotum (eg, lesions, cysts, rashes) • Epididymides (eg, size, symmetry, masses) • Testes (eg, size, symmetry, masses) • Urethral meatus (eg, size, location, lesions, discharge) • Penis (eg, lesions, presence or absence of foreskin, foreskin retractability, plaque, masses, scarring, deformities) Digital rectal examination including: • Prostate gland (eg, size, symmetry, nodularity, tenderness) • Seminal vesicles (eg, symmetry, tenderness, masses, enlargement) • Sphincter tone, presence of hemorrhoids, rectal masses

System/Body Area	Elements of Examination
Genitourinary (Cont'd)	**FEMALE:** Includes **at least seven of the following eleven** elements identified by bullets: • Inspection and palpation of breasts (eg, masses or lumps, tenderness, symmetry, nipple discharge) • Digital rectal examination including sphincter tone, presence of hemorrhoids, rectal masses Pelvic examination (with or without specimen collection for smears and cultures) including: • External genitalia (eg, general appearance, hair distribution, lesions) • Urethral meatus (eg, size, location, lesions, prolapse) • Urethra (eg, masses, tenderness, scarring) • Bladder (eg, fullness, masses, tenderness) • Vagina (eg, general appearance, estrogen effect, discharge, lesions, pelvic support, cystocele, rectocele) • Cervix (eg, general appearance, lesions, discharge) • Uterus (eg, size, contour, position, mobility, tenderness, consistency, descent or support) • Adnexa/parametria (eg, masses, tenderness, organomegaly, nodularity) • Anus and perineum
Lymphatic	• Palpation of lymph nodes in neck, axillae, groin and/or other location
Musculoskeletal	
Extremities	
Skin	• Inspection and/or palpation of skin and subcutaneous tissue (eg, rashes, lesions, ulcers)
Neurological/ Psychiatric	Brief assessment of mental status including • Orientation (eg, time, place and person) and • Mood and affect (eg, depression, anxiety, agitation)

Content and Documentation Requirements

Level of Exam	Perform and Document:
Problem Focused	**One to five** elements identified by a bullet.
Expanded Problem Focused	**At least six** elements identified by a bullet.
Detailed	**At least twelve** elements identified by a bullet.
Comprehensive	Perform **all** elements identified by a bullet; document every element in each box with a shaded border and at least one element in each box with an unshaded border.

Hematologic/Lymphatic/Immunologic Examination

System/Body Area	Elements of Examination
Constitutional	• Measurement of **any three of the following seven** vital signs: 1) sitting or standing blood pressure, 2) supine blood pressure, 3) pulse rate and regularity, 4) respiration, 5) temperature, 6) height, 7) weight (May be measured and recorded by ancillary staff) • General appearance of patient (eg, development, nutrition, body habitus, deformities, attention to grooming)
Head and Face	• Palpation and/or percussion of face with notation of presence or absence of sinus tenderness
Eyes	• Inspection of conjunctivae and lids
Ears, Nose, Mouth and Throat	• Otoscopic examination of external auditory canals and tympanic membranes • Inspection of nasal mucosa, septum and turbinates • Inspection of teeth and gums • Examination of oropharynx (eg, oral mucosa, hard and soft palates, tongue, tonsils, posterior pharynx)
Neck	• Examination of neck (eg, masses, overall appearance, symmetry, tracheal position, crepitus) • Examination of thyroid (eg, enlargement, tenderness, mass)
Respiratory	• Assessment of respiratory effort (eg, intercostal retractions, use of accessory muscles, diaphragmatic movement) • Auscultation of lungs (eg, breath sounds, adventitious sounds, rubs)
Cardiovascular	• Auscultation of heart with notation of abnormal sounds and murmurs • Examination of peripheral vascular system by observation (eg, swelling, varicosities) and palpation (eg, pulses, temperature, edema, tenderness)
Chest (Breasts)	
Gastrointestinal (Abdomen)	• Examination of abdomen with notation of presence of masses or tenderness • Examination of liver and spleen

System/Body Area	Elements of Examination
Genitourinary	
Lymphatic	• Palpation of lymph nodes in neck, axillae, groin, and/or other location
Musculoskeletal	
Extremities	• Inspection and palpation of digits and nails (eg, clubbing, cyanosis, inflammation, petechiae, ischemia, infections, nodes)
Skin	• Inspection and/or palpation of skin and subcutaneous tissue (eg, rashes, lesions, ulcers, ecchymoses, bruises)
Neurological/ Psychiatric	Brief assessment of mental status including • Orientation to time, place and person • Mood and affect (eg, depression, anxiety, agitation)

Content and Documentation Requirements

Level of Exam	Perform and Document:
Problem Focused	**One to five** elements identified by a bullet.
Expanded Problem Focused	**At least six** elements identified by a bullet.
Detailed	**At least twelve** elements identified by a bullet.
Comprehensive	Perform **all** elements identified by a bullet; document every element in each box with a shaded border and at least one element in each box with an unshaded border.

Musculoskeletal Examination

System/Body Area	Elements of Examination
Constitutional	• Measurement of **any three of the following seven** vital signs: 1) sitting or standing blood pressure, 2) supine blood pressure, 3) pulse rate and regularity, 4) respiration, 5) temperature, 6) height, 7) weight (May be measured and recorded by ancillary staff) • General appearance of patient (eg, development, nutrition, body habitus, deformities, attention to grooming)
Head and Face	
Eyes	
Ears, Nose, Mouth and Throat	
Neck	
Respiratory	
Cardiovascular	• Examination of peripheral vascular system by observation (eg, swelling, varicosities) and palpation (eg, pulses, temperature, edema, tenderness)
Chest (Breasts)	
Gastrointestinal (Abdomen)	
Genitourinary	
Lymphatic	• Palpation of lymph nodes in neck, axillae, groin and/or other location

System/Body Area	Elements of Examination
Musculoskeletal	• Examination of gait and station
	Examination of joint(s), bone(s) and muscle(s)/ tendon(s) of **four of the following six** areas: 1) head and neck; 2) spine, ribs and pelvis; 3) right upper extremity; 4) left upper extremity; 5) right lower extremity; and 6) left lower extremity. The examination of a given area includes: • Inspection, percussion and/or palpation with notation of any misalignment, asymmetry, crepitation, defects, tenderness, masses or effusions • Assessment of range of motion with notation of any pain (eg, straight leg raising), crepitation or contracture • Assessment of stability with notation of any dislocation (luxation), subluxation or laxity • Assessment of muscle strength and tone (eg, flaccid, cog wheel, spastic) with notation of any atrophy or abnormal movements NOTE: For the comprehensive level of examination, all four of the elements identified by a bullet must be performed and documented for each of four anatomic areas. For the three lower levels of examination, each element is counted separately for each body area. For example, assessing range of motion in two extremities constitutes two elements.
Extremities	[See musculoskeletal and skin]
Skin	• Inspection and/or palpation of skin and subcutaneous tissue (eg, scars, rashes, lesions, cafe-au-lait spots, ulcers) in **four of the following six** areas: 1) head and neck; 2) trunk; 3) right upper extremity; 4) left upper extremity; 5) right lower extremity; and 6) left lower extremity. NOTE: For the comprehensive level, the examination of all four anatomic areas must be performed and documented. For the three lower levels of examination, each body area is counted separately. For example, inspection and/or palpation of the skin and subcutaneous tissue of two extremitites constitutes two elements.

Neurological/ Psychiatric	• Test coordination (eg, finger/nose, heel/ knee/shin, rapid alternating movements in the upper and lower extremities, evaluation of fine motor coordination in young children)
	• Examination of deep tendon reflexes and/or nerve stretch test with notation of pathological reflexes (eg, Babinski)
	• Examination of sensation (eg, by touch, pin, vibration, proprioception)
	Brief assessment of mental status including
	• Orientation to time, place and person
	• Mood and affect (eg, depression, anxiety, agitation)

Content and Documentation Requirements

Level of Exam	Perform and Document:
Problem Focused	**One to five** elements identified by a bullet.
Expanded Problem Focused	**At least six** elements identified by a bullet.
Detailed	**At least twelve** elements identified by a bullet.
Comprehensive	Perform **all** elements identified by a bullet; document every element in each box with a shaded border and at least one element in each box with an unshaded border.

Neurological Examination

System/Body Area	Elements of Examination
Constitutional	• Measurement of **any three of the following seven** vital signs: 1) sitting or standing blood pressure, 2) supine blood pressure, 3) pulse rate and regularity, 4) respiration, 5) temperature, 6) height, 7) weight (May be measured and recorded by ancillary staff) • General appearance of patient (eg, development, nutrition, body habitus, deformities, attention to grooming)
Head and Face	
Eyes	• Ophthalmoscopic examination of optic discs (eg, size, C/D ratio, appearance) and posterior segments (eg, vessel changes, exudates, hemorrhages)
Ears, Nose, Mouth and Throat	
Neck	
Respiratory	
Cardiovascular	• Examination of carotid arteries (eg, pulse amplitude, bruits) • Auscultation of heart with notation of abnormal sounds and murmurs • Examination of peripheral vascular system by observation (eg, swelling, varicosities) and palpation (eg, pulses, temperature, edema, tenderness)
Chest (Breasts)	
Gastrointestinal (Abdomen)	
Genitourinary	
Lymphatic	

System/Body Area	Elements of Examination
Musculoskeletal	• Examination of gait and station Assessment of motor function including: • Muscle strength in upper and lower extremities • Muscle tone in upper and lower extremities (eg, flaccid, cog wheel, spastic) with notation of any atrophy or abnormal movements (eg, fasciculation, tardive dyskinesia)
Extremities	[See musculoskeletal]
Skin	
Neurological	Evaluation of higher integrative functions including: • Orientation to time, place and person • Recent and remote memory • Attention span and concentration • Language (eg, naming objects, repeating phrases, spontaneous speech) • Fund of knowledge (eg, awareness of current events, past history, vocabulary) Test the following cranial nerves: • 2nd cranial nerve (eg, visual acuity, visual fields, fundi) • 3rd, 4th and 6th cranial nerves (eg, pupils, eye movements) • 5th cranial nerve (eg, facial sensation, corneal reflexes) • 7th cranial nerve (eg, facial symmetry, strength) • 8th cranial nerve (eg, hearing with tuning fork, whispered voice and/or finger rub) • 9th cranial nerve (eg, spontaneous or reflex palate movement) • 11th cranial nerve (eg, shoulder shrug strength) • 12th cranial nerve (eg, tongue protrusion) • Examination of sensation (eg, by touch, pin, vibration, proprioception) • Examination of deep tendon reflexes in upper and lower extremities with notation of pathological reflexes (eg, Babinski) • Test coordination (eg, finger/nose, heel/knee/shin, rapid alternating movements in the upper and lower extremities, evaluation of fine motor coordination in young children)
Psychiatric	

Content and Documentation Requirements

Level of Exam	Perform and Document:
Problem Focused	**One to five** elements identified by a bullet.
Expanded Problem Focused	**At least six** elements identified by a bullet.
Detailed	**At least twelve** elements identified by a bullet.
Comprehensive	Perform **all** elements identified by a bullet; document every element in each box with a shaded border and at least one element in each box with an unshaded border.

Psychiatric Examination

System/Body Area	Elements of Examination
Constitutional	• Measurement of **any three of the following seven** vital signs: 1) sitting or standing blood pressure, 2) supine blood pressure, 3) pulse rate and regularity, 4) respiration, 5) temperature, 6) height, 7) weight (May be measured and recorded by ancillary staff) • General appearance of patient (eg, development, nutrition, body habitus, deformities, attention to grooming)
Head and Face	
Eyes	
Ears, Nose, Mouth and Throat	
Neck	
Respiratory	
Cardiovascular	
Chest (Breasts)	
Gastrointestinal (Abdomen)	
Genitourinary	
Lymphatic	
Musculoskeletal	• Assessment of muscle strength and tone (eg, flaccid, cog wheel, spastic) with notation of any atrophy and abnormal movements • Examination of gait and station
Extremities	
Skin	
Neurological	

System/Body Area	Elements of Examination
Psychiatric	• Description of speech including: rate; volume; articulation; coherence; and spontaneity with notation of abnormalities (eg, perseveration, paucity of language) • Description of thought processes including: rate of thoughts; content of thoughts (eg, logical vs. illogical, tangential); abstract reasoning; and computation • Description of associations (eg, loose, tangential, circumstantial, intact) • Description of abnormal or psychotic thoughts including: hallucinations; delusions; preoccupation with violence; homicidal or suicidal ideation; and obsessions • Description of the patient's judgment (eg, concerning everyday activities and social situations) and insight (eg, concerning psychiatric condition) Complete mental status examination including • Orientation to time, place and person • Recent and remote memory • Attention span and concentration • Language (eg, naming objects, repeating phrases) • Fund of knowledge (eg, awareness of current events, past history, vocabulary) • Mood and affect (eg, depression, anxiety, agitation, hypomania, lability)

Content and Documentation Requirements

Level of Exam	Perform and Document:
Problem Focused	**One to five** elements identified by a bullet.
Expanded Problem Focused	**At least six** elements identified by a bullet.
Detailed	**At least nine** elements identified by a bullet.
Comprehensive	Perform **all** elements identified by a bullet; document every element in each box with a shaded border and at least one element in each box with an unshaded border.

Respiratory Examination

System/Body Area	Elements of Examination
Constitutional	• Measurement of **any three of the following seven** vital signs: 1) sitting or standing blood pressure, 2) supine blood pressure, 3) pulse rate and regularity, 4) respiration, 5) temperature, 6) height, 7) weight (May be measured and recorded by ancillary staff) • General appearance of patient (eg, development, nutrition, body habitus, deformities, attention to grooming)
Head and Face	
Eyes	
Ears, Nose, Mouth and Throat	• Inspection of nasal mucosa, septum and turbinates • Inspection of teeth and gums • Examination of oropharynx (eg, oral mucosa, hard and soft palates, tongue, tonsils and posterior pharynx)
Neck	• Examination of neck (eg, masses, overall appearance, symmetry, tracheal position, crepitus) • Examination of thyroid (eg, enlargement, tenderness, mass) • Examination of jugular veins (eg, distension; a, v or cannon a waves)
Respiratory	• Inspection of chest with notation of symmetry and expansion • Assessment of respiratory effort (eg, intercostal retractions, use of accessory muscles, diaphragmatic movement) • Percussion of chest (eg, dullness, flatness, hyperresonance) • Palpation of chest (eg, tactile fremitus) • Auscultation of lungs (eg, breath sounds, adventitious sounds, rubs)
Cardiovascular	• Auscultation of heart including sounds, abnormal sounds and murmurs • Examination of peripheral vascular system by observation (eg, swelling, varicosities) and palpation (eg, pulses, temperature, edema, tenderness)
Chest (Breasts)	

System/Body Area	Elements of Examination
Gastrointestinal (Abdomen)	• Examination of abdomen with notation of presence of masses or tenderness • Examination of liver and spleen
Genitourinary	
Lymphatic	• Palpation of lymph nodes in neck, axillae, groin and/or other location
Musculoskeletal	• Assessment of muscle strength and tone (eg, flaccid, cog wheel, spastic) with notation of any atrophy and abnormal movements • Examination of gait and station
Extremities	• Inspection and palpation of digits and nails (eg, clubbing, cyanosis, inflammation, petechiae, ischemia, infections, nodes)
Skin	• Inspection and/or palpation of skin and subcutaneous tissue (eg, rashes, lesions, ulcers)
Neurological/ Psychiatric	Brief assessment of mental status including • Orientation to time, place and person • Mood and affect (eg, depression, anxiety, agitation)

Content and Documentation Requirements

Level of Exam	Perform and Document:
Problem Focused	**One to five** elements identified by a bullet.
Expanded Problem Focused	**At least six** elements identified by a bullet.
Detailed	**At least twelve** elements identified by a bullet.
Comprehensive	Perform **all** elements identified by a bullet; document every element in each box with a shaded border and at least one element in each box with an unshaded border.

Skin Examination

System/Body Area	Elements of Examination
Constitutional	• Measurement of any **three of the following seven** vital signs: 1) sitting or standing blood pressure, 2) supine blood pressure, 3) pulse rate and regularity, 4) respiration, 5) temperature, 6) height, 7) weight (May be measured and recorded by ancillary staff) • General appearance of patient (eg, development, nutrition, body habitus, deformities, attention to grooming)
Head and Face	
Eyes	• Inspection of conjunctivae and lids
Ears, Nose, Mouth and Throat	• Inspection of lips, teeth and gums • Examination of oropharynx (eg, oral mucosa, hard and soft palates, tongue, tonsils, posterior pharynx)
Neck	• Examination of thyroid (eg, enlargement, tenderness, mass)
Respiratory	
Cardiovascular	• Examination of peripheral vascular system by observation (eg, swelling, varicosities) and palpation (eg, pulses, temperature, edema, tenderness)
Chest (Breasts)	
Gastrointestinal (Abdomen)	• Examination of liver and spleen • Examination of anus for condyloma and other lesions
Genitourinary	
Lymphatic	• Palpation of lymph nodes in neck, axillae, groin and/or other location
Musculoskeletal	
Extremities	• Inspection and palpation of digits and nails (eg, clubbing, cyanosis, inflammation, petechiae, ischemia, infections, nodes)

System/Body Area	Elements of Examination
Skin	• Palpation of scalp and inspection of hair of scalp, eyebrows, face, chest, pubic area (when indicated) and extremities • Inspection and/or palpation of skin and subcutaneous tissue (eg, rashes, lesions, ulcers, susceptibility to and presence of photo damage) in **eight of the following ten** areas: • Head, including the face and • Neck • Chest, including breasts and axillae • Abdomen • Genitalia, groin, buttocks • Back • Right upper extremity • Left upper extremity • Right lower extremity • Left lower extremity NOTE: For the comprehensive level, the examination of at least eight anatomic areas must be performed and documented. For the three lower levels of examination, each body area is counted separately. For example, inspection and/or palpation of the skin and subcutaneous tissue of the right upper extremity and the left upper extremity constitutes two elements. • Inspection of eccrine and apocrine glands of skin and subcutaneous tissue with identification and location of any hyperhidrosis, chromhidroses or bromhidrosis
Neurological/ Psychiatric	Brief assessment of mental status including • Orientation to time, place and person • Mood and affect (eg, depression, anxiety, agitation)

Content and Documentation Requirements

Level of Exam	Perform and Document:
Problem Focused	**One to five** elements identified by a bullet.
Expanded Problem Focused	**At least six** elements identified by a bullet.
Detailed	**At least twelve** elements identified by a bullet.
Comprehensive	Perform **all** elements identified by a bullet; document every element in each box with a shaded border and at least one element in each box with an unshaded border.

C. DOCUMENTATION OF THE COMPLEXITY OF MEDICAL DECISION MAKING

The levels of E/M services recognize four types of medical decision making (straight-forward, low complexity, moderate complexity and high complexity). Medical decision making refers to the complexity of establishing a diagnosis and/or selecting a management option as measured by:

- the number of possible diagnoses and/or the number of management options that must be considered;

- the amount and/or complexity of medical records, diagnostic tests, and/or other information that must be obtained, reviewed and analyzed; and

- the risk of significant complications, morbidity and/or mortality, as well as comorbidities, associated with the patient's presenting problem(s), the diagnostic procedure(s) and/or the possible management options.

The chart below shows the progression of the elements required for each level of medical decision making. To qualify for a given type of decision making, **two of the three elements in the table must be either met or exceeded.**

Number of diagnoses or management options	Amount and/or complexity of data to be reviewed	Risk of complications and/or morbidity or mortality	Type of decision making
Minimal	Minimal or None	Minimal	*Straightforward*
Limited	Limited	Low	*Low Complexity*
Multiple	Moderate	Moderate	*Moderate Complexity*
Extensive	Extensive	High	*High Complexity*

Each of the elements of medical decision making is described below.

43

NUMBER OF DIAGNOSES OR MANAGEMENT OPTIONS

The number of possible diagnoses and/or the number of management options that must be considered is based on the number and types of problems addressed during the encounter, the complexity of establishing a diagnosis and the management decisions that are made by the physician.

Generally, decision making with respect to a diagnosed problem is easier than that for an identified but undiagnosed problem. The number and type of diagnostic tests employed may be an indicator of the number of possible diagnoses. Problems which are improving or resolving are less complex than those which are worsening or failing to change as expected. The need to seek advice from others is another indicator of complexity of diagnostic or management problems.

> ●*DG:* *For each encounter, an assessment, clinical impression, or diagnosis should be documented. It may be explicitly stated or implied in documented decisions regarding management plans and/or further evaluation.*
>
> > • *For a presenting problem with an established diagnosis the record should reflect whether the problem is: a) improved, well controlled, resolving or resolved; or, b) inadequately controlled, worsening, or failing to change as expected.*
> >
> > • *For a presenting problem without an established diagnosis, the assessment or clinical impression may be stated in the form of differential diagnoses or as a "possible", "probable", or "rule out" (R/O) diagnosis.*
>
> ●*DG:* *The initiation of, or changes in, treatment should be documented. Treatment includes a wide range of management options including patient instructions, nursing instructions, therapies, and medications.*
>
> ●*DG:* *If referrals are made, consultations requested or advice sought, the record should indicate to whom or where the referral or consultation is made or from whom the advice is requested.*

AMOUNT AND/OR COMPLEXITY OF DATA TO BE REVIEWED

The amount and complexity of data to be reviewed is based on the types of diagnostic testing ordered or reviewed. A decision to obtain and review old medical records and/or obtain history from sources other than the patient increases the amount and complexity of data to be reviewed.

Discussion of contradictory or unexpected test results with the physician who performed or interpreted the test is an indication of the complexity of data being reviewed. On occasion the physician who ordered a test may personally review the image, tracing or specimen to supplement information from the physician who prepared the test report or interpretation; this is another indication of the complexity of data being reviewed.

●*DG: If a diagnostic service (test or procedure) is ordered, planned, scheduled, or performed at the time of the E/M encounter, the type of service, eg, lab or x-ray, should be documented.*

●*DG: The review of lab, radiology and/or other diagnostic tests should be documented. A simple notation such as "WBC elevated" or "chest x-ray unremarkable" is acceptable. Alternatively, the review may be documented by initialing and dating the report containing the test results.*

●*DG: A decision to obtain old records or decision to obtain additional history from the family, caretaker or other source to supplement that obtained from the patient should be documented.*

●*DG: Relevant findings from the review of old records, and/or the receipt of additional history from the family, caretaker or other source to supplement that obtained from the patient should be documented. If there is no relevant information beyond that already obtained, that fact should be documented. A notation of "Old records reviewed" or "additional history obtained from family" without elaboration is insufficient.*

●*DG: The results of discussion of laboratory, radiology or other diagnostic tests with the physician who performed or interpreted the study should be documented.*

●*DG: The direct visualization and independent interpretation of an image, tracing or specimen previously or subsequently interpreted by another physician should be documented.*

RISK OF SIGNIFICANT COMPLICATIONS, MORBIDITY, AND/OR MORTALITY

The risk of significant complications, morbidity, and/or mortality is based on the risks associated with the presenting problem(s), the diagnostic procedure(s), and the possible management options.

> ●*DG: Comorbidities/underlying diseases or other factors that increase the complexity of medical decision making by increasing the risk of complications, morbidity, and/or mortality should be documented.*

> ●*DG: If a surgical or invasive diagnostic procedure is ordered, planned or scheduled at the time of the E/M encounter, the type of procedure, eg, laparoscopy, should be documented.*

> ●*DG: If a surgical or invasive diagnostic procedure is performed at the time of the E/M encounter, the specific procedure should be documented.*

> ●*DG: The referral for or decision to perform a surgical or invasive diagnostic procedure on an urgent basis should be documented or implied.*

The following table may be used to help determine whether the risk of significant complications, morbidity, and/or mortality is *minimal*, *low*, *moderate*, or *high*. Because the determination of risk is complex and not readily quantifiable, the table includes common clinical examples rather than absolute measures of risk. The assessment of risk of the presenting problem(s) is based on the risk related to the disease process anticipated between the present encounter and the next one. The assessment of risk of selecting diagnostic procedures and management options is based on the risk during and immediately following any procedures or treatment. **The highest level of risk in any one category (presenting problem(s), diagnostic procedure(s), or management options) determines the overall risk.**

TABLE OF RISK

Level of Risk	Presenting Problem(s)	Diagnostic Procedure(s) Ordered	Management Options Selected
Minimal	• One self-limited or minor problem, eg, cold, insect bite, tinea corporis	• Laboratory tests requiring venipuncture • Chest x-rays • EKG/EEG • Urinalysis • Ultrasound, eg, echocardiography • KOH prep	• Rest • Gargles • Elastic bandages • Superficial dressings
Low	• Two or more self-limited or minor problems • One stable chronic illness, eg, well controlled hypertension, non-insulin dependent diabetes, cataract, BPH • Acute uncomplicated illness or injury, eg, cystitis, allergic rhinitis, simple sprain	• Physiologic tests not under stress, eg, pulmonary function tests • Non-cardiovascular imaging studies with contrast, eg, barium enema • Superficial needle biopsies • Clinical laboratory tests requiring arterial puncture • Skin biopsies	• Over-the-counter drugs • Minor surgery with no identified risk factors • Physical therapy • Occupational therapy • IV fluids without additives
Moderate	• One or more chronic illnesses with mild exacerbation, progression, or side effects of treatment • Two or more stable chronic illnesses • Undiagnosed new problem with uncertain prognosis, eg, lump in breast • Acute illness with systemic symptoms, eg, pyelonephritis, pneumonitis, colitis • Acute complicated injury, eg, head injury with brief loss of consciousness	• Physiologic tests under stress, eg, cardiac stress test, fetal contraction stress test • Diagnostic endoscopies with no identified risk factors • Deep needle or incisional biopsy • Cardiovascular imaging studies with contrast and no identified risk factors, eg, arteriogram, cardiac catheterization • Obtain fluid from body cavity, eg lumbar puncture, thoracentesis, culdocentesis	• Minor surgery with identified risk factors • Elective major surgery (open, percutaneous or endoscopic) with no identified risk factors • Prescription drug management • Therapeutic nuclear medicine • IV fluids with additives • Closed treatment of fracture or dislocation without manipulation
High	• One or more chronic illnesses with severe exacerbation, progression, or side effects of treatment • Acute or chronic illnesses or injuries that pose a threat to life or bodily function, eg, multiple trauma, acute MI, pulmonary embolus, severe respiratory distress, progressive severe rheumatoid arthritis, psychiatric illness with potential threat to self or others, peritonitis, acute renal failure • An abrupt change in neurologic status, eg, seizure, TIA, weakness, sensory loss	• Cardiovascular imaging studies with contrast with identified risk factors • Cardiac electrophysiological tests • Diagnostic Endoscopies with identified risk factors • Discography	• Elective major surgery (open, percutaneous or endoscopic) with identified risk factors • Emergency major surgery (open, percutaneous or endoscopic) • Parenteral controlled substances • Drug therapy requiring intensive monitoring for toxicity • Decision not to resuscitate or to de-escalate care because of poor prognosis

D. DOCUMENTATION OF AN ENCOUNTER DOMINATED BY COUNSELING OR COORDINATION OF CARE

In the case where counseling and/or coordination of care dominates (more than 50%) of the physician/patient and/or family encounter (face-to-face time in the office or other or outpatient setting, floor/unit time in the hospital or nursing facility), time is considered the key or controlling factor to qualify for a particular level of E/M services.

> ●*DG: If the physician elects to report the level of service based on counseling and/or coordination of care, the total length of time of the encounter (face-to-face or floor time, as appropriate) should be documented and the record should describe the counseling and/or activities to coordinate care.*

1995 Documentation Guidelines for Evaluation and Management Services

Source: _Documentation Guidelines for Evaluation and Management Services,_ ©1995. _American Medical Association,_
http://www.hcfa.gov/medicare/mcarpti.htm

1995 DOCUMENTATION GUIDELINES
FOR EVALUATION & MANAGEMENT SERVICES

I. INTRODUCTION

WHAT IS DOCUMENTATION AND WHY IS IT IMPORTANT?

Medical record documentation is required to record pertinent facts, findings, and observations about an individual's health history including past and present illnesses, examinations, tests, treatments, and outcomes. The medical record chronologically documents the care of the patient and is an important element contributing to high quality care. The medical record facilitates:

- the ability of the physician and other health care professionals to evaluate and plan the patient's immediate treatment, and to monitor his/her health care over time.

- communication and continuity of care among physicians and other health care professionals involved in the patient's care;

- accurate and timely claims review and payment;

- appropriate utilization review and quality of care evaluations; and

- collection of data that may be useful for research and education.

An appropriately documented medical record can reduce many of the "hassles" associated with claims processing and may serve as a legal document to verify the care provided, if necessary.

WHAT DO PAYERS WANT AND WHY?

Because payers have a contractual obligation to enrollees, they may require reasonable documentation that services are consistent with the insurance coverage provided. They may request information to validate:

- the site of service;

- the medical necessity and appropriateness of the diagnostic and/or therapeutic services provided; and/or

- that services provided have been accurately reported.

II. GENERAL PRINCIPLES OF MEDICAL RECORD DOCUMENTATION

The principles of documentation listed below are applicable to all types of medical and surgical services in all settings. For Evaluation and Management (E/M) services, the nature and amount of physician work and documentation varies by type of service, place of service and the patient's status. The general principles listed below may be modified to account for these variable circumstances in providing E/M services.

1. The medical record should be complete and legible.

2. The documentation of each patient encounter should include:

    •   reason for the encounter and relevant history, physical examination findings and prior diagnostic test results;

    •   assessment, clinical impression or diagnosis;

    •   plan for care; and

    •   date and legible identity of the observer.

3. If not documented, the rationale for ordering diagnostic and other ancillary services should be easily inferred.

4. Past and present diagnoses should be accessible to the treating and/or consulting physician.

5. Appropriate health risk factors should be identified.

6. The patient's progress, response to and changes in treatment, and revision of diagnosis should be documented.

7. The CPT and ICD-9-CM codes reported on the health insurance claim form or billing statement should be supported by the documentation in the medical record.

3/4/99 1:36pm

III.   DOCUMENTATION OF E/M SERVICES

This publication provides definitions and documentation guidelines for the three *key* components of E/M services and for visits which consist predominately of counseling or coordination of care. The three key components--history, examination, and medical decision making--appear in the descriptors for office and other outpatient services, hospital observation services, hospital inpatient services, consultations, emergency department services, nursing facility services, domiciliary care services, and home services. While some of the text of CPT has been repeated in this publication, the reader should refer to CPT for the complete descriptors for E/M services and instructions for selecting a level of service. **Documentation guidelines are identified by the symbol *DG* .**

The descriptors for the levels of E/M services recognize seven components which are used in defining the levels of E/M services. These components are:

- history;
- examination;
- medical decision making;
- counseling;
- coordination of care;
- nature of presenting problem; and
- time.

The first three of these components (i.e., history, examination and medical decision making) are the *key* components in selecting the level of E/M services. An exception to this rule is the case of visits which consist predominantly of counseling or coordination of care; for these services time is the key or controlling factor to qualify for a particular level of E/M service.

For certain groups of patients, the recorded information may vary slightly from that described here. Specifically, the medical records of infants, children, adolescents and pregnant women may have additional or modified information recorded in each history and examination area.

As an example, newborn records may include under history of the present illness (HPI) the details of mother's pregnancy and the infant's status at birth; social history will focus on family structure; family history will focus on congenital anomalies and hereditary disorders in the family. In addition, information on growth and development and/or nutrition will be recorded. Although not specifically defined in these documentation guidelines, these patient group variations on history and examination are appropriate.

A.   DOCUMENTATION OF HISTORY

The levels of E/M services are based on four types of history (Problem Focused, Expanded Problem Focused, Detailed, and Comprehensive.) Each type of history includes some or all of the following elements:

- Chief complaint (CC);

- History of present illness (HPI);

- Review of systems (ROS); and

- Past, family and/or social history (PFSH).

The extent of history of present illness, review of systems and past, family and/or social history that is obtained and documented is dependent upon clinical judgement and the nature of the presenting problem(s).

The chart below shows the progression of the elements required for each type of history. To qualify for a given type of history, **all three elements in the table must be met.** (A chief complaint is indicated at all levels.)

History of Present Illness (HPI)	Review of Systems (ROS)	Past, Family, and/or Social History (PFSH)	Type of History
Brief	N/A	N/A	*Problem Focused*
Brief	Problem Pertinent	N/A	*Expanded Problem Focused*
Extended	Extended	Pertinent	*Detailed*
Extended	Complete	Complete	*Comprehensive*

●*DG: The CC, ROS and PFSH may be listed as separate elements of history, or they may be included in the description of the history of the present illness.*

●*DG:* *A ROS and/or a PFSH obtained during an earlier encounter does not need to be re-recorded if there is evidence that the physician reviewed and updated the previous information. This may occur when a physician updates his or her own record or in an institutional setting or group practice where many physicians use a common record. The review and update may be documented by:*

- *describing any new ROS and/or PFSH information or noting there has been no change in the information; and*

- *noting the date and location of the earlier ROS and/or PFSH.*

●*DG:* *The ROS and/or PFSH may be recorded by ancillary staff or on a form completed by the patient. To document that the physician reviewed the information, there must be a notation supplementing or confirming the information recorded by others.*

●*DG:* *If the physician is unable to obtain a history from the patient or other source, the record should describe the patient's condition or other circumstance which precludes obtaining a history.*

Definitions and specific documentation guidelines for each of the elements of history are listed below.

CHIEF COMPLAINT (CC)

The CC is a concise statement describing the symptom, problem, condition, diagnosis, physician recommended return, or other factor that is the reason for the encounter.

●*DG:* *The medical record should clearly reflect the chief complaint.*

HISTORY OF PRESENT ILLNESS (HPI)

The HPI is a chronological description of the development of the patient's present illness from the first sign and/or symptom or from the previous encounter to the present. It includes the following elements:

- location,
- quality,
- severity,
- duration,
- timing,
- context,
- modifying factors, and
- associated signs and symptoms.

Brief and *extended* HPIs are distinguished by the amount of detail needed to accurately characterize the clinical problem(s).

A *brief* HPI consists of one to three elements of the HPI.

> ●*DG: The medical record should describe one to three elements of the present illness (HPI).*

An *extended* HPI consists of four or more elements of the HPI.

> ●*DG: The medical record should describe four or more elements of the present illness (HPI) or associated comorbidities.*

3/4/99 1:36pm

REVIEW OF SYSTEMS (ROS)

A ROS is an inventory of body systems obtained through a series of questions seeking to identify signs and/or symptoms which the patient may be experiencing or has experienced.

For purposes of ROS, the following systems are recognized:

- Constitutional symptoms (e.g., fever, weight loss)
- Eyes
- Ears, Nose, Mouth, Throat
- Cardiovascular
- Respiratory
- Gastrointestinal
- Genitourinary
- Musculoskeletal
- Integumentary (skin and/or breast)
- Neurological
- Psychiatric
- Endocrine
- Hematologic/Lymphatic
- Allergic/Immunologic

A *problem pertinent* ROS inquires about the system directly related to the problem(s) identified in the HPI.

> ●*DG:* *The patient's positive responses and pertinent negatives for the system related to the problem should be documented.*

An *extended* ROS inquires about the system directly related to the problem(s) identified in the HPI and a limited number of additional systems.

> ●*DG:* *The patient's positive responses and pertinent negatives for two to nine systems should be documented.*

A *complete* ROS inquires about the system(s) directly related to the problem(s) identified in the HPI <u>plus</u> all additional body systems.

> ●*DG:* *At least ten organ systems must be reviewed. Those systems with positive or pertinent negative responses must be individually documented. For the remaining systems, a notation indicating all other systems are negative is permissible. In the absence of such a notation, at least ten systems must be individually documented.*

3/4/99 1:36pm

PAST, FAMILY AND/OR SOCIAL HISTORY (PFSH)

The PFSH consists of a review of three areas:

- past history (the patient's past experiences with illnesses, operations, injuries and treatments);

- family history (a review of medical events in the patient's family, including diseases which may be hereditary or place the patient at risk); and

- social history (an age appropriate review of past and current activities).

For the categories of subsequent hospital care, follow-up inpatient consultations and subsequent nursing facility care, CPT requires only an "interval" history. It is not necessary to record information about the PFSH.

A *pertinent* PFSH is a review of the history area(s) directly related to the problem(s) identified in the HPI.

> ●*DG:* *At least one specific item from* <u>*any*</u> *of the three history areas must be documented for a pertinent PFSH .*

A **complete** PFSH is of a review of two or all three of the PFSH history areas, depending on the category of the E/M service. A review of all three history areas is required for services that by their nature include a comprehensive assessment or reassessment of the patient. A review of two of the three history areas is sufficient for other services.

> ●*DG* *At least one specific item from* <u>*two*</u> *of the three history areas must be documented for a complete PFSH for the following categories of E/M services: office or other outpatient services, established patient; emergency department; subsequent nursing facility care; domiciliary care, established patient; and home care, established patient.*

> ●*DG:* *At least one specific item from* <u>*each*</u> *of the three history areas must be documented for a complete PFSH for the following categories of E/M services: office or other outpatient services, new patient; hospital observation services; hospital inpatient services, initial care; consultations; comprehensive nursing facility assessments; domiciliary care, new patient; and home care, new patient.*

B. DOCUMENTATION OF EXAMINATION

The levels of E/M services are based on four types of examination that are defined as follows:

- *Problem Focused* -- a limited examination of the affected body area or organ system.

- *Expanded Problem Focused* -- a limited examination of the affected body area or organ system and other symptomatic or related organ system(s).

- *Detailed* -- an extended examination of the affected body area(s) and other symptomatic or related organ system(s).

- *Comprehensive* -- a general multi-system examination or complete examination of a single organ system.

For purposes of examination, the following *body areas* are recognized:

- Head, including the face
- Neck
- Chest, including breasts and axillae
- Abdomen
- Genitalia, groin, buttocks
- Back, including spine
- Each extremity

For purposes of examination, the following *organ systems* are recognized:

- Constitutional (e.g., vital signs, general appearance)
- Eyes
- Ears, nose, mouth and throat
- Cardiovascular
- Respiratory
- Gastrointestinal
- Genitourinary
- Musculoskeletal
- Skin
- Neurologic
- Psychiatric
- Hematologic/lymphatic/immunologic

The extent of examinations performed and documented is dependent upon clinical judgement and the nature of the presenting problem(s). They range from limited examinations of single body areas to general multi-system or complete single organ system examinations.

> ●DG: *Specific abnormal and relevant negative findings of the examination of the affected or symptomatic body area(s) or organ system(s) should be documented. A notation of "abnormal" without elaboration is insufficient.*

> ●DG: *Abnormal or unexpected findings of the examination of the unaffected or asymptomatic body area(s) or organ system(s) should be described.*

> ●DG: *A brief statement or notation indicating "negative" or "normal" is sufficient to document normal findings related to unaffected area(s) or asymptomatic organ system(s).*

> ●DG: *The medical record for a general multi-system examination should include findings about 8 or more of the 12 organ systems.*

C. DOCUMENTATION OF THE COMPLEXITY OF MEDICAL DECISION MAKING

The levels of E/M services recognize four types of medical decision making (straight-forward, low complexity, moderate complexity and high complexity). Medical decision making refers to the complexity of establishing a diagnosis and/or selecting a management option as measured by:

- the number of possible diagnoses and/or the number of management options that must be considered;

- the amount and/or complexity of medical records, diagnostic tests, and/or other information that must be obtained, reviewed and analyzed; and

- the risk of significant complications, morbidity and/or mortality, as well as comorbidities, associated with the patient's presenting problem(s), the diagnostic procedure(s) and/or the possible management options.

3/4/99 1:36pm

The chart below shows the progression of the elements required for each level of medical decision making. To qualify for a given type of decision making two of the three elements in the table must be either met or exceeded.

Number of diagnoses or management options	Amount and/or complexity of data to be reviewed	Risk of complications and/or morbidity or mortality	Type of decision making
Minimal	Minimal or None	Minimal	*Straightforward*
Limited	Limited	Low	*Low Complexity*
Multiple	Moderate	Moderate	*Moderate Complexity*
Extensive	Extensive	High	*High Complexity*

Each of the elements of medical decision making is described below.

NUMBER OF DIAGNOSES OR MANAGEMENT OPTIONS

The number of possible diagnoses and/or the number of management options that must be considered is based on the number and types of problems addressed during the encounter, the complexity of establishing a diagnosis and the management decisions that are made by the physician.

Generally, decision making with respect to a diagnosed problem is easier than that for an identified but undiagnosed problem. The number and type of diagnostic tests employed may be an indicator of the number of possible diagnoses. Problems which are improving or resolving are less complex than those which are worsening or failing to change as expected. The need to seek advice from others is another indicator of complexity of diagnostic or management problems.

> ●*DG:* *For each encounter, an assessment, clinical impression, or diagnosis should be documented. It may be explicitly stated or implied in documented decisions regarding management plans and/or further evaluation.*
>
> - *For a presenting problem with an established diagnosis the record should reflect whether the problem is: a) improved, well controlled, resolving or resolved; or, b) inadequately controlled, worsening, or failing to change as expected.*
>
> - *For a presenting problem without an established diagnosis, the assessment or clinical impression may be stated in the form of a differential diagnoses or as "possible", "probable", or "rule out" (R/O) diagnoses.*

3/4/99 1:36pm

- *DG: The initiation of, or changes in, treatment should be documented. Treatment includes a wide range of management options including patient instructions, nursing instructions, therapies, and medications.*

- *DG: If referrals are made, consultations requested or advice sought, the record should indicate to whom or where the referral or consultation is made or from whom the advice is requested.*

AMOUNT AND/OR COMPLEXITY OF DATA TO BE REVIEWED

The amount and complexity of data to be reviewed is based on the types of diagnostic testing ordered or reviewed. A decision to obtain and review old medical records and/or obtain history from sources other than the patient increases the amount and complexity of data to be reviewed.

Discussion of contradictory or unexpected test results with the physician who performed or interpreted the test is an indication of the complexity of data being reviewed. On occasion the physician who ordered a test may personally review the image, tracing or specimen to supplement information from the physician who prepared the test report or interpretation; this is another indication of the complexity of data being reviewed.

- *DG: If a diagnostic service (test or procedure) is ordered, planned, scheduled, or performed at the time of the E/M encounter, the type of service, eg, lab or x-ray, should be documented.*

- *DG: The review of lab, radiology and/or other diagnostic tests should be documented. An entry in a progress note such as "WBC elevated" or "chest x-ray unremarkable" is acceptable. Alternatively, the review may be documented by initialing and dating the report containing the test results.*

- *DG: A decision to obtain old records or decision to obtain additional history from the family, caretaker or other source to supplement that obtained from the patient should be documented.*

- *DG: Relevant finding from the review of old records, and/or the receipt of additional history from the family, caretaker or other source should be documented. If there is no relevant information beyond that already obtained, that fact should be documented. A notation of "Old records reviewed" or "additional history obtained from family" without elaboration is insufficient.*

3/4/99 1:36pm

DG: *The results of discussion of laboratory, radiology or other diagnostic tests with the physician who performed or interpreted the study should be documented.*

DG: *The direct visualization and independent interpretation of an image, tracing or specimen previously or subsequently interpreted by another physician should be documented.*

RISK OF SIGNIFICANT COMPLICATIONS, MORBIDITY, AND/OR MORTALITY

The risk of significant complications, morbidity, and/or mortality is based on the risks associated with the presenting problem(s), the diagnostic procedure(s), and the possible management options.

DG: *Comorbidities/underlying diseases or other factors that increase the complexity of medical decision making by increasing the risk of complications, morbidity, and/or mortality should be documented.*

DG: *If a surgical or invasive diagnostic procedure is ordered, planned or scheduled at the time of the E/M encounter, the type of procedure, eg, laparoscopy, should be documented.*

DG: *If a surgical or invasive diagnostic procedure is performed at the time of the E/M encounter, the specific procedure should be documented.*

DG: *The referral for or decision to perform a surgical or invasive diagnostic procedure on an urgent basis should be documented or implied.*

The following table may be used to help determine whether the risk of significant complications, morbidity, and/or mortality is *minimal*, *low*, *moderate*, or *high*. Because the determination of risk is complex and not readily quantifiable, the table includes common clinical examples rather than absolute measures of risk. The assessment of risk of the presenting problem(s) is based on the risk related to the disease process anticipated between the present encounter and the next one. The assessment of risk of selecting diagnostic procedures and management options is based on the risk during and immediately following any procedures or treatment. The highest level of risk in any one category (presenting problem(s), diagnostic procedure(s), or management options) determines the overall risk.

TABLE OF RISK

Level of Risk	Presenting Problem(s)	Diagnostic Procedure(s) Ordered	Management Options Selected
Minimal	• One self-limited or minor problem, eg cold, insect bite, tinea corporis	• Laboratory tests requiring venipuncture • Chest x-rays • EKG/EEG • Urinalysis • Ultrasound, eg, echocardiography • KOH prep	• Rest • Gargles • Elastic bandages • Superficial dressings
Low	• Two or more self-limited or minor problems • One stable chronic illness, eg well controlled hypertension or non-insulin dependent diabetes, cataract, BPH • Acute uncomplicated illness or injury, eg, cystitis, allergic rhinitis, simple sprain	• Physiologic tests not under stress, eg, pulmonary function tests • Non-cardiovascular imaging studies with contrast, eg, barium enema • Superficial needle biopsies • Clinical laboratory tests requiring arterial puncture • Skin biopsies	• Over-the-counter drugs • Minor surgery with no identified risk factors • Physical therapy • Occupational therapy • IV fluids without additives
Moderate	• One or more chronic illnesses with mild exacerbation, progression, or side effects of treatment • Two or more stable chronic illnesses • Undiagnosed new problem with uncertain prognosis, eg, lump in breast • Acute illness with systemic symptoms, eg, pyelonephritis, pneumonitis, colitis • Acute complicated injury, eg head injury with brief loss of consciousness	• Physiologic tests under stress, eg, cardiac stress test, fetal contraction stress test • Diagnostic endoscopies with no identified risk factors • Deep needle or incisional biopsy • Cardiovascular imaging studies with contrast and no identified risk factors, eg arteriogram, cardiac catheterization • Obtain fluid from body cavity, eg lumbar puncture, thoracentesis, culdocentesis	• Minor surgery with identified risk factors • Elective major surgery (open, percutaneous or endoscopic) with no identified risk factors • Prescription drug management • Therapeutic nuclear medicine • IV fluids with additives • Closed treatment of fracture or dislocation without manipulation
High	• One or more chronic illnesses with severe exacerbation, progression, or side effects of treatment • Acute or chronic illnesses or injuries that pose a threat to life or bodily function, eg multiple trauma, acute MI, pulmonary embolus, severe respiratory distress, progressive severe rheumatoid arthritis, psychiatric illness with potential threat to self or others, peritonitis, acute renal failure • An abrupt change in neurologic status, eg seizure, TIA, weakness, or sensory loss	• Cardiovascular imaging studies with contrast with identified risk factors • Cardiac electrophysiological tests • Diagnostic Endoscopies with identified risk factors • Discography	• Elective major surgery (open, percutaneous or endoscopic) with identified risk factors • Emergency major surgery (open, percutaneous or endoscopic) • Parenteral controlled substances • Drug therapy requiring intensive monitoring for toxicity • Decision not to resuscitate or to de-escalate care because of poor prognosis

D. DOCUMENTATION OF AN ENCOUNTER DOMINATED BY COUNSELING OR COORDINATION OF CARE

In the case where counseling and/or coordination of care dominates (more than 50%) of the physician/patient and/or family encounter (face-to-face time in the office or other outpatient setting or floor/unit time in the hospital or nursing facility), time is considered the key or controlling factor to qualify for a particular level of E/M services.

> ●*DG: If the physician elects to report the level of service based on counseling and/or coordination of care, the total length of time of the encounter (face-to-face or floor time, as appropriate) should be documented and the record should describe the counseling and/or activities to coordinate care.*

Appendix E

Glossary

Appeal request — The request for a review by a Medicare provider who questions the correctness of reimbursement for services rendered.

Assignment — When a provider accepts the Medicare approved amount as payment in full, it is called accepting assignment. In most cases, Medicare pays 80 percent and the beneficiary pays the 20 percent co-payment.

Balanced Budget Act of 1997 — Legislation signed by President Clinton on August 5, 1997, significantly changing the Medicare program. The legislation expanded the opportunities for nurse practitioner (NP) and clinical nurse specialist (CNS) direct reimbursement by the Medicare program and expanded Medicare coverage to some preventive services.

Beneficiary — The person who is entitled to Medicare benefits under the Social Security Act.

Capitation — A set amount of money per patient received or paid out to the provider for a defined period of time that covers contracted services and is paid in advance of the delivery of the service.

Claim — The request for payment of professional fees for services provided to the beneficiary.

Coding — The process of documenting and communicating to the Medicare carrier the services performed and the diagnostic conditions treated, using a standardized listing of alphanumeric codes.

Co-payment — The fixed portion of the claim or expense that the beneficiary is responsible for paying the provider of the services.

Current Procedural Terminology (CPT) — System for coding professional services developed by the American Medical Association to file claims with Medicare and other third-party payers.

Department of Health and Human Services (HHS) — Department within the U.S. government that is responsible for administering health and social welfare programs.

Durable medical equipment (DME) — Medical equipment that is not disposable and is related to care for a medical condition. It is equipment that is intended to be used again and again, such as a wheelchair or a hospital bed.

Diagnoses-Related Groups (DRGs) — A statistical system for classifying any inpatient stay into groups for purposes of Part A Medicare payments. This system is the basis of reimbursement that Medicare uses to pay hospitals for Medicare beneficiaries.

Evaluation and management (E&M) services — Patient evaluation and management services that a health professional provides during a patient's office visit, hospital stay, or other visit or consultation.

Fee-for-service — A reimbursement method in which the providers charge for each professional service or unit provided to the beneficiary.

Health Care Financing Administration (HCFA) — The federal agency within the Department of Health and Human Services (HHS) that oversees all aspects of health financing for the Medicare program.

HCFA Common Procedure Coding System (HCPCS) — Coding system required for billing Medicare that describes services and procedures. HCPCS includes Current Procedural Terminology (CPT) but also has codes for services not included in CPT, such as durable medical equipemnt (DME) and ambulance services.

International Classification of Diseases, 9th revision, clinical modification (ICD-9-CM) — The classification of disease by diagnosis codified into alphanumeric codes to enable providers to effectively document the medical condition, symptom, or complaint that is the basis for providing the service.

Medicaid — A federal and state medical assistance program that provides basic health benefits for persons who meet the eligibility requirements for their state Medicaid program.

Medicare — A federal health care program for people age 65 years or older and for people with conditions such as end-stage renal disease. Coverage includes Part A, inpatient hospital services, and Part B, outpatient physician services.

Medicare carriers — Health insurance companies that enter into a contract with the Health Care Financing Administration (HCFA) to serve as the administrative contractor to process and adjudicate claims under the Medicare Part B outpatient health program for beneficiaries in a defined geographical area.

Medicare intermediaries — Insurance companies that have contracts with the Health Care Financing Administration (HCFA) to process claims under Part A (hospital insurance) of Medicare.

Medicare managed care — A healthcare plan option beneficiaries can select to receive their Medicare benefits. Managed care plans have contracts with the Health Care Financing Administration (HCFA) to provide Medicare benefits. When a beneficiary enrolls in a Medicare managed care plan, he or she chooses a primary care provider from the plan's panel of primary care providers. This primary care provider is then responsible for coordinating all of the health care services for the beneficiary.

Medicare fee schedule — A payment schedule adopted by the Health Care Financing Administration (HCFA) for payment of Part B services based on the resource cost of professional work, practice overhead, and professional liability insurance, with adjustments for differences in geographical location. The fee schedule indicates the maximum Medicare payment for the service for participating and nonparticipating providers as well as a fee schedule for clinical laboratory tests and durable medical equipment.

Medicare supplement — Private insurance coverage that pays for the services not covered by the Medicare program.

Part B Premium — A monthly premium paid by the Medicare beneficiary to cover Part B services in fee-for-service Medicare. Members of Medicare managed care plans must also pay this premium to receive full coverage and to be eligible to enroll and stay in the managed care plan.

Participating provider — A provider who signs a participation contract, agreeing to accept assignment on all claims submitted to Medicare for processing.

Provider — A generic term for any person or entity approved to provide or to give care to Medicare beneficiaries and to receive payment from Medicare.

Resource-Based Relative Value Scale (RBRVS) — A relative value scale based on the resource costs of providing Part B Medicare services.

Review — A request for additional consideration by Medicare of a previously processed service.

Upcoding — The practice of a provider billing for a procedure that pays better than the service actually provided.